AF711841

TABLE OF CONTENTS

Secret Key #1 - Time is Your Greatest Enemy

Pace Yourself

Wear a watch. At the beginning of the test, check the time (or start a chronometer on your watch to count the minutes), and check the time after every few questions to make sure you are "on schedule."

If you are forced to speed up, do it efficiently. Usually one or more answer choices can be eliminated without too much difficulty. Above all, don't panic. Don't speed up and just begin guessing at random choices. By pacing yourself, and continually monitoring your progress against your watch, you will always know exactly how far ahead or behind you are with your available time. If you find that you are one minute behind on the test, don't skip one question without spending any time on it, just to catch back up. Take 15 fewer seconds on the next four questions, and after four questions you'll have caught back up. Once you catch back up, you can continue working each problem at your normal pace.

Furthermore, don't dwell on the problems that you were rushed on. If a problem was taking up too much time and you made a hurried guess, it must be difficult. The difficult questions are the ones you are most likely to miss anyway, so it isn't a big loss. It is better to end with more time than you need than to run out of time.

Lastly, sometimes it is beneficial to slow down if you are constantly getting ahead of time. You are always more likely to catch a careless mistake by working more slowly than quickly, and among very high-scoring test takers (those who are likely to have lots of time left over), careless errors affect the score more than mastery of material.

Secret Key #2 - Guessing is not Guesswork

You probably know that guessing is a good idea - unlike other standardized tests, there is no penalty for getting a wrong answer. Even if you have no idea about a question, you still have a 20-25% chance of getting it right.

Most test takers do not understand the impact that proper guessing can have on their score. Unless you score extremely high, guessing will significantly contribute to your final score.

Monkeys Take the Test

What most test takers don't realize is that to insure that 20-25% chance, you have to guess randomly. If you put 20 monkeys in a room to take this test, assuming they answered once per question and behaved themselves, on average they would get 20-25% of the questions correct. Put 20 test takers in the room, and the average will be much lower among guessed questions. Why?

1. The test writers intentionally writes deceptive answer choices that "look" right. A test taker has no idea about a question, so picks the "best looking" answer, which is often wrong. The monkey has no idea what looks good and what doesn't, so will consistently be lucky about 20-25% of the time.
2. Test takers will eliminate answer choices from the guessing pool based on a hunch or intuition. Simple but correct answers often get excluded, leaving a 0% chance of being correct. The monkey has no clue, and often gets lucky with the best choice.

This is why the process of elimination endorsed by most test courses is flawed and detrimental to your performance- test takers don't guess, they make an ignorant stab in the dark that is usually worse than random.

$5 Challenge

Let me introduce one of the most valuable ideas of this course- the $5 challenge:

You only mark your "best guess" if you are willing to bet $5 on it.

You only eliminate choices from guessing if you are willing to bet $5 on it.

Why $5? Five dollars is an amount of money that is small yet not insignificant, and can really add up fast (20 questions could cost you $100). Likewise, each answer choice on one question of the test will have a small impact on your overall score, but it can really add up to a lot of points in the end.

The process of elimination IS valuable. The following shows your chance of guessing it right:

If you eliminate wrong answer choices until only this many answer choices remain:	1	2	3
Chance of getting it correct:	100%	50%	33%

However, if you accidentally eliminate the right answer or go on a hunch for an incorrect answer, your chances drop dramatically: to 0%. By guessing among all the answer choices, you are GUARANTEED to have a shot at the right answer.

That's why the $5 test is so valuable- if you give up the advantage and safety of a pure guess, it had better be worth the risk.

What we still haven't covered is how to be sure that whatever guess you make is truly random. Here's the easiest way:

Always pick the first answer choice among those remaining.

Such a technique means that you have decided, **before you see a single test question**, exactly how you are going to guess- and since the order of choices tells you nothing about which one is correct, this guessing technique is perfectly random.

This section is not meant to scare you away from making educated guesses or eliminating choices- you just need to define when a choice is worth eliminating. The $5 test, along with a pre-defined random guessing strategy, is the best way to make sure you reap all of the benefits of guessing.

Secret Key #3 - Practice Smarter, Not Harder

Many test takers delay the test preparation process because they dread the awful amounts of practice time they think necessary to succeed on the test. We have refined an effective method that will take you only a fraction of the time.

There are a number of "obstacles" in your way to succeed. Among these are answering questions, finishing in time, and mastering test-taking strategies. All must be executed on the day of the test at peak performance, or your score will suffer. The test is a mental marathon that has a large impact on your future.

Just like a marathon runner, it is important to work your way up to the full challenge. So first you just worry about questions, and then time, and finally strategy:

Success Strategy

1. Find a good source for practice tests.
2. If you are willing to make a larger time investment, consider using more than one study guide- often the different approaches of multiple authors will help you "get" difficult concepts.
3. Take a practice test with no time constraints, with all study helps "open book." Take your time with questions and focus on applying strategies.
4. Take a practice test with time constraints, with all guides "open book."
5. Take a final practice test with no open material and time limits

If you have time to take more practice tests, just repeat step 5. By gradually exposing yourself to the full rigors of the test environment, you will condition your mind to the stress of test day and maximize your success.

Secret Key #4 - Prepare, Don't Procrastinate

Let me state an obvious fact: if you take the test three times, you will get three different scores. This is due to the way you feel on test day, the level of preparedness you have, and, despite the test writers' claims to the contrary, some tests WILL be easier for you than others.

Since your future depends so much on your score, you should maximize your chances of success. In order to maximize the likelihood of success, you've got to prepare in advance. This means taking practice tests and spending time learning the information and test taking strategies you will need to succeed.

Never take the test as a "practice" test, expecting that you can just take it again if you need to. Feel free to take sample tests on your own, but when you go to take the official test, be prepared, be focused, and do your best the first time!

Secret Key #5 - Test Yourself

Everyone knows that time is money. There is no need to spend too much of your time or too little of your time preparing for the test. You should only spend as much of your precious time preparing as is necessary for you to get the score you need.

Once you have taken a practice test under real conditions of time constraints, then you will know if you are ready for the test or not.

If you have scored extremely high the first time that you take the practice test, then there is not much point in spending countless hours studying. You are already there.

Benchmark your abilities by retaking practice tests and seeing how much you have improved. Once you score high enough to guarantee success, then you are ready.

If you have scored well below where you need, then knuckle down and begin studying in earnest. Check your improvement regularly through the use of practice tests under real conditions. Above all, don't worry, panic, or give up. The key is perseverance!

Then, when you go to take the test, remain confident and remember how well you did on the practice tests. If you can score high enough on a practice test, then you can do the same on the real thing.

Top 20 Test Taking Tips

1. Carefully follow all the test registration procedures
2. Know the test directions, duration, topics, question types, how many questions
3. Setup a flexible study schedule at least 3-4 weeks before test day
4. Study during the time of day you are most alert, relaxed, and stress free
5. Maximize your learning style; visual learner use visual study aids, auditory learner use auditory study aids
6. Focus on your weakest knowledge base
7. Find a study partner to review with and help clarify questions
8. Practice, practice, practice
9. Get a good night's sleep; don't try to cram the night before the test
10. Eat a well balanced meal
11. Know the exact physical location of the testing site; drive the route to the site prior to test day
12. Bring a set of ear plugs; the testing center could be noisy
13. Wear comfortable, loose fitting, layered clothing to the testing center; prepare for it to be either cold or hot during the test
14. Bring at least 2 current forms of ID to the testing center
15. Arrive to the test early; be prepared to wait and be patient
16. Eliminate the obviously wrong answer choices, then guess the first remaining choice
17. Pace yourself; don't rush, but keep working and move on if you get stuck
18. Maintain a positive attitude even if the test is going poorly
19. Keep your first answer unless you are positive it is wrong
20. Check your work, don't make a careless mistake

General Strategies

The most important thing you can do is to ignore your fears and jump into the test immediately- do not be overwhelmed by any strange-sounding terms. You have to jump into the test like jumping into a pool- all at once is the easiest way.

Make Predictions

As you read and understand the question, try to guess what the answer will be. Remember that several of the answer choices are wrong, and once you begin reading them, your mind will immediately become cluttered with answer choices designed to throw you off. Your mind is typically the most focused immediately after you have read the question and digested its contents. If you can, try to predict what the correct answer will be. You may be surprised at what you can predict.

Quickly scan the choices and see if your prediction is in the listed answer choices. If it is, then you can be quite confident that you have the right answer. It still won't hurt to check the other answer choices, but most of the time, you've got it!

Answer the Question

It may seem obvious to only pick answer choices that answer the question, but the test writers can create some excellent answer choices that are wrong. Don't pick an answer just because it sounds right, or you believe it to be true. It MUST answer the question. Once you've made your selection, always go back and check it against the question and make sure that you didn't misread the question, and the answer choice does answer the question posed.

Benchmark

After you read the first answer choice, decide if you think it sounds correct or not. If it doesn't, move on to the next answer choice. If it does, mentally mark that answer choice. This doesn't mean that you've definitely selected it as your answer choice, it just means that it's the best you've seen thus far. Go ahead and read the next choice. If the next choice is worse than the one you've already selected, keep going to the next answer choice. If the next choice is better than the choice you've already selected, mentally mark the new answer choice as your best guess.

The first answer choice that you select becomes your standard. Every other answer choice must be benchmarked against that standard. That choice is correct until proven otherwise by another answer choice beating it out. Once you've decided that no other answer choice seems as good, do one final check to ensure that your answer choice answers the question posed.

Valid Information

Don't discount any of the information provided in the question. Every piece of information may be necessary to determine the correct answer. None of the information in the question is there to throw you off (while the answer choices will certainly have information to throw you off). If two seemingly unrelated topics are discussed, don't ignore either. You can be confident there is a relationship, or it wouldn't be included in the question, and you are probably going to have to determine what is that relationship to find the answer.

Avoid "Fact Traps"

Don't get distracted by a choice that is factually true. Your search is for the answer that answers the question. Stay focused and don't fall for an answer that is true but incorrect. Always go back to the question and make sure you're choosing an answer that actually answers the question and is not just a true statement. An answer can be factually correct, but it MUST answer the question asked. Additionally, two answers can both be seemingly correct, so be sure to read all of the answer choices, and make sure that you get the one that BEST answers the question.

Milk the Question

Some of the questions may throw you completely off. They might deal with a subject you have not been exposed to, or one that you haven't reviewed in years. While your lack of knowledge about the subject will be a hindrance, the question itself can give you many clues that will help you find the correct answer. Read the question carefully and look for clues. Watch particularly for adjectives and nouns describing difficult terms or words that you don't recognize. Regardless of if you completely understand a word or not, replacing it with a synonym either provided or one you more familiar with may help you to understand what the questions are asking. Rather than wracking your mind about specific detailed information concerning a difficult term or word, try to use mental substitutes that are easier to understand.

The Trap of Familiarity

Don't just choose a word because you recognize it. On difficult questions, you may not recognize a number of words in the answer choices. The test writers don't put "make-believe" words on the test; so don't think that just because you only recognize all the words in one answer choice means that answer choice must be correct. If you only recognize words in one answer choice, then focus on that one. Is it correct? Try your best to determine if it is correct. If it is, that is great, but if it doesn't, eliminate it. Each word and answer choice you eliminate increases your chances of getting the question correct, even if you then have to guess among the unfamiliar choices.

Eliminate Answers

Eliminate choices as soon as you realize they are wrong. But be careful! Make sure you consider all of the possible answer choices. Just because one appears right, doesn't mean that the next one won't be even better! The test writers will usually put more than one good answer choice for every question, so read all of them. Don't worry if you are stuck between two that seem right. By getting down to just two remaining possible choices, your odds are now 50/50. Rather than wasting too much time, play the odds. You are guessing, but guessing wisely, because you've been able to knock out some of the answer choices that you know are wrong. If you are eliminating choices and realize that the last answer choice you are left with is also obviously wrong, don't panic. Start over and consider each choice again. There may easily be something that you missed the first time and will realize on the second pass.

Tough Questions

If you are stumped on a problem or it appears too hard or too difficult, don't waste time. Move on! Remember though, if you can quickly check for obviously incorrect answer choices, your chances of guessing correctly are greatly improved. Before you completely give up, at least try to knock out a couple of possible answers. Eliminate what you can and then guess at the remaining answer choices before moving on.

Brainstorm

If you get stuck on a difficult question, spend a few seconds quickly brainstorming. Run through the complete list of possible answer choices. Look at each choice and ask yourself, "Could this answer the question satisfactorily?" Go through each answer choice and consider it independently of the other. By systematically going through all possibilities, you may find something that you would otherwise overlook. Remember that when you get stuck, it's important to try to keep moving.

Read Carefully

Understand the problem. Read the question and answer choices carefully. Don't miss the question because you misread the terms. You have plenty of time to read each question thoroughly and make sure you understand what is being asked. Yet a happy medium must be attained, so don't waste too much time. You must read carefully, but efficiently.

Face Value

When in doubt, use common sense. Always accept the situation in the problem at face value. Don't read too much into it. These problems will not require you to make huge leaps of logic. The test writers aren't trying to throw you off with a cheap trick. If you have to go beyond creativity and make a leap of logic in order to have an answer choice answer the question, then you should look at the other answer choices. Don't overcomplicate the problem by creating theoretical relationships or explanations that will warp time or space. These are normal problems rooted in reality. It's just that the applicable relationship or explanation may not be readily apparent and you have to figure things out. Use your common sense to interpret anything that isn't clear.

Prefixes

If you're having trouble with a word in the question or answer choices, try dissecting it. Take advantage of every clue that the word might include. Prefixes and suffixes can be a huge help. Usually they allow you to determine a basic meaning. Pre- means before, post- means after, pro - is positive, de- is negative. From these prefixes and suffixes, you can get an idea of the general meaning of the word and try to put it into context. Beware though of any traps. Just because con is the opposite of pro, doesn't necessarily mean congress is the opposite of progress!

Hedge Phrases

Watch out for critical "hedge" phrases, such as likely, may, can, will often, sometimes, often, almost, mostly, usually, generally, rarely, sometimes. Question writers insert these hedge phrases to cover every possibility. Often an answer choice will be wrong simply because it leaves no room for exception. Avoid answer choices that have definitive words like "exactly," and "always".

Switchback Words

Stay alert for "switchbacks". These are the words and phrases frequently used to alert you to shifts in thought. The most common switchback word is "but". Others include although, however, nevertheless, on the other hand, even though, while, in spite of, despite, regardless of.

New Information

Correct answer choices will rarely have completely new information included. Answer choices typically are straightforward reflections of the material asked about and will directly relate to the question. If a new piece of information is included in an answer choice that doesn't even seem to relate to the topic being asked about, then that answer choice is likely incorrect. All of the information needed to answer the question is usually provided for you, and so you should not have to make guesses that are unsupported or choose answer choices that require unknown information that cannot be reasoned on its own.

Time Management

On technical questions, don't get lost on the technical terms. Don't spend too much time on any one question. If you don't know what a term means, then since you don't have a dictionary, odds are you aren't going to get much further. You should immediately recognize terms as whether or not you know them. If you don't, work with the other clues that you have, the other answer choices and terms provided, but don't waste too much time trying to figure out a difficult term.

Contextual Clues

Look for contextual clues. An answer can be right but not correct. The contextual clues will help you find the answer that is most right and is correct. Understand the context in which a phrase or statement is made. This will help you make important distinctions.

Don't Panic

Panicking will not answer any questions for you. Therefore, it isn't helpful. When you first see the question, if your mind goes blank, take a deep breath. Force yourself to mechanically go through the steps of solving the problem and using the strategies you've learned.

Pace Yourself

Don't get clock fever. It's easy to be overwhelmed when you're looking at a page full of questions, your mind is full of random thoughts and feeling confused, and the clock is ticking down faster than you would like. Calm down and maintain the pace that you have set for yourself. As long as you are on track by monitoring your pace, you are guaranteed to have enough time for yourself. When you get to the last few minutes of the test, it may seem like you won't have enough time left, but if you only have as many questions as you should have left at that point, then you're right on track!

Answer Selection

The best way to pick an answer choice is to eliminate all of those that are wrong, until only one is left and confirm that is the correct answer. Sometimes though, an answer choice may immediately look right. Be careful! Take a second to make sure that the other choices are not equally obvious. Don't make a hasty mistake. There are only two times that you should stop before checking other answers. First is when you are positive that the answer choice you have selected is correct. Second is when time is almost out and you have to make a quick guess!

Check Your Work

Since you will probably not know every term listed and the answer to every question, it is important that you get credit for the ones that you do know. Don't miss any questions through careless mistakes. If at all possible, try to take a second to look back over your answer selection and make sure you've selected the correct answer choice and haven't made a costly careless mistake (such as marking an answer choice that you didn't mean to mark). This quick double check should more than pay for itself in caught mistakes for the time it costs.

Beware of Directly Quoted Answers

Sometimes an answer choice will repeat word for word a portion of the question or reference section. However, beware of such exact duplication – it may be a trap! More than likely, the correct choice will paraphrase or summarize a point, rather than being exactly the same wording.

Slang

Scientific sounding answers are better than slang ones. An answer choice that begins "To compare the outcomes…" is much more likely to be correct than one that begins "Because some people insisted…"

Extreme Statements

Avoid wild answers that throw out highly controversial ideas that are proclaimed as established fact. An answer choice that states the "process should used in certain situations, if…" is much more likely to be correct than one that states the "process should be discontinued completely." The first is a calm rational statement and doesn't even make a definitive, uncompromising stance, using a hedge word "if" to provide wiggle room, whereas the second choice is a radical idea and far more extreme.

Answer Choice Families

When you have two or more answer choices that are direct opposites or parallels, one of them is usually the correct answer. For instance, if one answer choice states "x increases" and another answer choice states "x decreases" or "y increases," then those two or three answer choices are very similar in construction and fall into the same family of answer choices. A family of answer choices is when two or three answer choices are very similar in construction, and yet often have a directly opposite meaning. Usually the correct answer choice will be in that family of answer choices. The "odd man out" or answer choice that doesn't seem to fit the parallel construction of the other answer choices is more likely to be incorrect.

Be Aware of the Following Hints

1. 350 questions offered given on the NBDHE test. The first part of the exam covers 200 questions:

I. Scientific Basis for Dental Hygiene Practice

II. Provision of Clinical Dental Hygiene Services

III. Community Health Activities

2. The second part of the exam is 150 questions based on case scenarios.
3. The NBDHE is offered on paper.

Bones of the head

Skull

The bones of an adult are joined (sutured) to protect the brain, and the eyes, and to form the nasal passages. The occipital bone is the posterior bone with a foramen which allows the nerves of the spinal cord to reach the brain. The lateral parts of this bone join the first vertebra of the spine. The frontal bone forms the upper part of the forehead, the area around the eyes and the eyebrows. This bone joins the parietal and temporal bones to form the sides of the head and the face. The sphenoid bone is at the center of the skull and extends to the other bones of the skull to support the nerves and blood vessels that supply the face, teeth, tongue, eyes, and ears. The ethmoid is a single bone that houses the nasal cavity and the sinuses.

Face

The maxilla forms the roof of the mouth and contains sinuses, the zygomatic process (or cheek bone), frontal process, palatine process, and orbital process. They join the bones that give them their names, the infraorbital foramen which allows the maxillary nerve to reach the maxillary teeth, and the maxillary tuberosity immediately behind the maxillary third molar. The maxillary tuberosity contains the posterior superior alveolar foramina that allows the superior alveolar nerves, veins, and arteries to reach the maxillary teeth and gingival.

Temporomandibular joint

The TMJ is the joint of the temporal bone with the condyle of the mandible. Working properly, it allows the mandible to move forward, to move backward, to move up and down, and to move side to side. The meniscus or fibrous disc, which looks like a doughnut of tendon with a thin membrane covering the doughnut hole moves between synovial fluid under the temporal fossa and floats on synovial fluid at the top of the condyle, cushions both bones. It can tear or become displaced and cause pain. Sometimes malocclusion of the teeth can put strain on the muscles that control the TMJ and cause pain or damage. Congenital malformations, bone degeneration caused by arthritis, or tumors also cause dysfunction.

Muscles

Mastication

Muscles of mastication are those that enable the person to open and close, and perform other movements of the mandible. This allows the person to speak, and to swallow food after he/she chews, or masticates, his/her food. These muscles receive sensation and "orders" from the brain through the motor branch of the trigeminal (V3) nerve. The *temporalis* muscle is shaped like a fan reaching from the floor of the temporal fossa to the coronoid process of the mandible. The *masseter* muscle is attached to the zygomatic arch and to the angle and bottom of the ramus. *Medial* and *lateral pterygoid* muscles originate on the lateral pterygoid plate and the superior head of the sphenoid bone. They attach at the angle of the mandible. These muscles must work together like a well-practiced orchestra if the mandible is to raise, lower, and move side to side smoothly.

Muscles of facial expressions

The muscles that allow facial expressions are attached to various bones and to the soft tissues of the face. They exchange information through the facial nerve (CN VII). The *orbicularis oris* circles the mouth and purses the lips. The term *depressor* refers to lowering action; *anguli* refers to an angle, *oris* refers to the mouth and *labii* refers to lips. Therefore *depressor labii inferioris* depresses the angle of the lower lip. *Mentalis* refers to the chin. The *buccinator muscle* pulls the lip to the side and helps to keep food on the occlusal surface of the teeth while chewing. *Risoris muscle* widens the mouth. *Levator labii superioris alaeque nasi muscles* raise the upper lip and the ala of the nose. *Zygomaticus major* and *minor* raises the angle of the mouth. *Platysma* pulls down the mouth and raises the skin of the neck. *Orbicularis oculi, corrugator supercilii*, and *frontal belly of epicranius muscles* close the eyelid, cause frown lines, and raise the eyebrows.

Nerves

Five branches of the maxillary branch of the trigeminal nerve

The posterior superior alveolar branch goes through the posterior superior alveolar foramina to the third molar and facial gingiva, the second molar and facial gingiva, and the palatal and distobuccal root of the first molar and the facial gingiva. The middle superior alveolar branch provides sensation to the mesiobuccal root of the first molar, the second premolar, and the first premolar. The anterior superior alveolar branch provides sensation to the cuspid and the lateral and central incisors. The posterior palatine branch provides sensation to the palatal gingiva of the molars and premolars (greater palatine), and the lesser palatine branch serves the soft palate. The anterior palatine (nasopalatine) branch serves the palatal gingiva of the anterior teeth.

Three branches of the mandibular branch of the trigeminal nerve

The mandibular branch is composed of the anterior trunk (buccal nerve and muscular branches) and the posterior trunk (auriculotemporal, lingual, and inferior alveolar nerves).The inferior alveolar nerve follows the mandibular canal before forming two further branches – the incisive nerve spreads into branches that provide sensation to the mandibular anterior teeth and around the periodontium. The mental nerve separates from the incisive nerve and exits the mandibular canal at the mental foramen. It forms branches to provide sensation to the facial gingiva of the mandibular anterior teeth, the chin, the lower lip, and the labial mucosa. The buccal nerve provides sensation to the facial gingiva of the mandibular molars and premolars. The lingual nerve provides sensation to the floor of the mouth, the tongue, and the mandibular lingual gingiva

Arteries and veins

The vascular system provides nutrients to the body. The subclavian and common carotid arteries provide most of the nutrition to the head, and the internal and external jugular veins drain the same area. The most reliable pulse is found at the carotid sinus about a finger width below the angle of the jaw. Most of the blood supply to the brain goes through the two anterior right and left internal carotid arteries, entering through the carotid canals, and through the two posterior vertebral arteries that go through the foramen magnum. These four arteries form the circle of Willis. The veins follow a path similar to the arteries to get to the brain. Unlike the veins in the rest of the body, the veins of the head and neck do not have valves to prevent backflow; therefore, they are not as resistant to infections as others.

Tissues

The body is made of several types of tissue which contain components with different functions. Tissues contain cells, intercellular substance such as collagen, and fluids. Tissue fluid in plasma carries nutrients to the rest of the body. Epithelial tissues cover or line surfaces, or form specialized structures such as tooth enamel and salivary glands. They depend on connective tissue for nutrition. Connective tissues can be loose, dense, cartilage, bone, or fluid. They support, hydrate, and bind other tissues together in addition to carrying nutrients. Muscle tissues are specialized. They can be voluntarily controlled to move arms and/or legs, or they can work involuntarily to make the heart pump. Muscle tissues are classified as skeletal (connected to the skeleton), smooth (in the intestines) or cardiac (heart).

Nerve tissue is divided into the soft, fragile central nervous system (brain and spinal cord) and the tougher, peripheral nervous system which sensitizes the rest of the body.

Dentition development

Primary dentition begins eruption at about 8 months with the mandibular central incisors erupting prior to maxillary centrals. Lateral incisors erupt at about 11 – 13 months followed by primary first molars at about 16 months. Primary canines (cuspids) erupt at about 19 – 20 months, and primary second molars are usually present by 24 – 29 months.

The permanent dentition begins erupting at about 6. Lateral incisors follow the central incisors and first molars at about 7 – 8 years. First and second premolars and cuspids erupt in that order between 10 and 12 years of age. Generally, eruption of the permanent dentition follows the same pattern and timetable as the eruption of the primary dentition. Second molars usually erupt at about 12 years, and third molars erupt at about 17. The third molars (wisdom teeth) may be partially erupted/impacted or congenitally missing.

Primary and permanent morphology

Primary teeth allow the child to learn to chew solid food, and they hold the position in the jaw for the same permanent teeth, with the exception of the molars. Primary molars hold the position for permanent premolars or bicuspids. The jaw grows to accommodate permanent molars. Primary teeth are shaped much like the permanent teeth and are designed for the same functions. Incisors are shaped like chisels to cut into food. Cuspids are designed for tearing food, and molars are intended to allow crushing. Primary teeth also support the facial muscles and soft tissues. Incisors, laterals, cuspids have one root as a general rule. Mandibular molars have two roots and maxillary molars usually have three roots. The crowns have whiter enamel and due to constriction at the CEJ, more bulbous curves

Permanent teeth replace exfoliated primary teeth. The teeth grow toward the deciduous teeth and cause the roots to dissolve as they get close. As the unerupted incisor develops, the developmental lobes flatten to form a shallow fossa on the lingual/palatal surface. The lobes, more obvious on erupted cuspids, flatten somewhat leaving two fossae with a lingual ridge separating them and a cingulum at the gingival margin where the lobes join. Centrals, laterals, and cuspids have one root. The canines, with longer roots than other teeth, are considered "cornerstones" of the face.

Mandibular premolars have two cusps and one root. Maxillary first premolars usually have two roots fused for the length of the root. Maxillary second premolars have one root, sometimes two. Permanent molars have four cusps, with an assortment of occlusal grooves corresponding to four developmental lobes. The maxillary molars usually have a palatal root, a mesiobuccal root and a distobuccal root.

Occlusion

Occlusion not only refers to the relationship of the mandibular arch with the maxillary arch, it refers to the relationship of the teeth within the arch. Developing occlusion is affected by surrounding muscles, the nerves, and the TMJ. Occlusion must be considered during treatment planning because it can contribute to various dental problems. Concentric occlusion refers to the habitual position of the teeth as the person tries to find the maximum contact and equal force on the teeth. Angle's Classification of Malocclusion is the usual occlusal classification standard. Class I is considered ideal and has the mesiobuccal cusp of the permanent maxillary first molar resting in the buccal groove of the mandibular first molar and the permanent maxillary cuspid resting between the mandibular canine and the first molar.

Malocclusion

Malocclusion can cause trauma to permanent teeth or to the TMJ. Crowded teeth hinder good oral hygiene and can cause periodontal disease. Overbite and overjet refer to the relationship of the maxillary incisors with the mandibular incisors. Severe overbite can cause trauma to the maxilla and damage to the condyle of the mandible. Class II, Division I, according to Angle's classification, presents the mesiobuccal cusp of the maxillary first molar forward of the buccal groove of the mandibular first molar and the cuspid forward of the mandibular cuspid with maxillary incisors extending toward the facial. Class II, Division II is the same as Division I except that the maxillary incisors lean toward the tongue. Class III presents with the maxillary first molar distal to the mandibular first molar and the maxillary cuspid distal to the mandibular cuspid by about half the width of a premolar.

Enamel and cementum

Enamel is the hardest substance in the body and consists of 96% inorganic matter and 4% organic matter. It covers the crown of the tooth and joins the cementum at the cementoenamel junction (CEJ). Ameloblasts, which come from ectodermal tissue, form enamel of hydroxyapatite crystals of calcium phosphate in a matrix of rods, rod sheaths, and interrod substance.

The cementum is 50% organic and 50% inorganic. It covers the dentin in the root of the tooth to provide an attachment surface for the periodontal ligament. Cementoblasts, located in the PDL, form collagen fibers and hydroxyapatite in the matrix. Cementum is both acellular, in the apical half, and cellular, in the cervical half. The outer surface of cementum, the cementoid, is hypocalcified; it contains Sharpey's fibers of PDL that embed in the cementoid.

Dentin and pulp

Dentin is the middle layer of the tooth and consists of 70% inorganic and 30% organic matter. The first part of the tooth to mineralize, it is formed from dental papilla by odontoblasts. It contains collagen and hydroxyapatite crystals. Dentinal tubules form a matrix from the DEJ to the pulp and contain nerve fibers for sensation. Throughout the life of the tooth secondary or reparative dentin can form in response to trauma or caries. Sclerotic dentin forms when the odontoblasts degenerate and the tubules fill with calcium salt. If the odontoblasts die but the tubule does not fill with calcium salt, the tooth dies.
The pulp is the non-mineralized portion of the tooth which develops from the dental papilla. It contains the nerves and the blood supply. Fibroblasts maintain the pulp tissue while histocytes and undifferentiated mesenchymal cells defend against disease. Korff's fibers form the dentinal matrix and odontoblasts repair it.

Periodontal ligament

Periodontal ligament (PDL) is a specialized connective tissue that attaches the cementum of the tooth to the bone. Though it produces cementum and lamina dura, it does not calcify. The fibrils of the ligament are made by fibroblasts, and collagen makes up the fibrils. Sharpey's fibers consist of different types of connective fibers. Free gingival fibers connect the gingiva to the tooth. Transseptal fibers connect the mesial surface to the distal surface of adjacent teeth. Alveolar crest fibers help resist horizontal movement by connecting the alveolar crest to the cementum. Horizontal fibers resist horizontal pressure by connecting cementum to the bone, and apical fibers surround the apex of the tooth to connect it to the bone. Oblique fibers prevent the apex of the tooth from being jammed into the socket by connecting obliquely from the bone toward the crown. Interradicular fibers help stabilize multi-rooted teeth by connecting multiple roots and bone.

Alveolar bone

Alveolar bone, 50% organic and 50% inorganic, surrounds and supports teeth. Compact bone, the cortical plate, is the outside wall of the mandible and the maxilla. Trabecular, spongy, bone makes the inside wall of the mandible and the maxilla. Red bone marrow forms blood (hemopoiesis) and yellow bone marrow consists of fatty tissue (which does not produce blood). Together they fill the spaces around the trabeculae. The periosteum covers the outside of the bone, and the endosteum covers the inside. Osteoblasts cells form bone, and osteocytes are osteoblasts that are trapped inside the bone and maintain contact with adjacent osteocytes. Canaliculi connect lacunae (the space occupied by osteocytes). The lamellae, thin layers of mature bone, consist of circumferential bone (the outer layer) and subendosteal (the surface of trabeculaer) bone. The Haversian system consists of the Haversian canal which carries tiny blood vessels and Volkmann's canal through which the blood vessels pass.

Gingiva

Gingiva contains fibrous connective tissue and stratified squamous epithelial tissues and attaches to the underlying bone. The sulcus, the space between the gingiva and the tooth, surrounds the tooth and ends at the epithelial attachment to the tooth. Free gingiva refers to the gingiva that is not attached to the tooth; the free gingival groove denotes sulcus depth. The mucogingival junction is the layer between the gingiva and the bone where the attached gingiva ends.

Tooth development

Oral epithelium (ectoderm) thickens to form the dental lamina, and the tooth germ begins to grow from the lamina into the underlying tissue (mesoderm). The enamel organ forms enamel, then the dental papilla forms dentin and pulp. Finally the dental sac forms the PDL, cementum and lamina dura. The enamel organ contains low cuboidal cells in the outer epithelium, star-shaped epithelial cells (stellate reticulum), flat epithelial cells (stratum intermedium), and cuboidal cells in the inner enamel epithelium. The basement membrane separates the enamel organ from the dental papilla and becomes the DEJ. As the enamel organ compresses, it produces the reduced enamel epithelium to protect the tooth until it erupts. The enamel cuticle forms; then the Hertwig epithelial root sheath, which produces dentin and determines the shape of the dentin and the number of roots, forms. The rests of Malassez (remnants of Hertwig's epithelial root sheath) form the PDL.

Oral mucous membrane

Three forms of mucosa form the oral mucous membrane. Masticatory mucosa is keratinized and includes the gingiva and the hard palate. Nonkeratinized mucosa forms the lining of the cheeks, soft palate, and the ventral surface of the tongue. Specialized mucosa includes the papillae and the top of the tongue. The oral mucous membrane protects the oral structures, secretes moisture to maintain the surface texture, and absorbs nutrients.

Circulatory system

Circulatory system consists of the heart, the blood vessels (veins, arteries, and capillaries), and the blood. The heart pumps the blood through the arteries, capillaries, and veins throughout the body picking up oxygen from the lungs, nutrients from the digestive system, and taking carbon dioxide and cellular wastes to the lungs or the kidneys. The arteries are specifically designed with thick, elastic walls to transport oxygenated blood away from the heart to smaller arterioles. Capillary walls are thin so that oxygen and nutrients can pass through them for use by the cells and so that waste products can be sent away for removal. The veins also have thin walls, and some have one-way valves to prevent blood from flowing back. The veins of the head and neck do not have these valves. Most of the veins carry un-oxygenated blood back to the heart then to the lungs for more oxygen.

The heart

The heart is specialized, involuntary cardiac muscle enclosed in pericardial membrane. The myocardium (muscular layer) and the endocardium (lining) keep the muscle tissue moist to facilitate movement. The right atrium receives blood from the superior and inferior vena cavae. Blood flows through the tricuspid valve into the right ventricle which sends it through the pulmonary valve and the pulmonary artery to the lungs. The left atrium receives oxygenated blood through four pulmonary veins and sends it into the left ventricle through the mitral valve. The left ventricle pumps arterial blood into the rest of the body through the aortic valve and the aorta. The heart is controlled by its own electrical system consisting of the sinoatrial node (pacemaker) and the atrioventricular node. The sinoatrial node controls the contraction of the atria and signals the atrioventricular node to tell the ventricles to contract. At the end of this cycle, the heart rests.

Blood function

The heart and blood vessels maintain body temperature at about 98.6°F, blood pressure at about 120/80 mmHg, glucose concentration at about 0.1% and pH at about 7.4. The blood supplies oxygen and nutrients to cells and removes carbon dioxide and wastes. It sends white blood cells to attack infections and hormones to various organs. It provides clotting factors when a blood vessel breaks and carries heat away from working muscles.

Red blood cells (erythrocytes), formed in bone marrow, contain hemoglobin to carry oxygen and number about 4 to 6 million per cubic mm of blood. White blood cells (leukocytes), about 5,000 to 11,000 per cubic mm of blood, are formed in bone marrow to fight infections by surrounding bacteria. Lymphocytes are agranular WBCs responsible for immunity. Platelets, about 150,000 to 300,000 per cubic mm, are the clotting factor. Plasma, the liquid part of blood, includes hormones, gasses, plasma proteins, salts, and nutrients.

Respiratory system function

The respiratory system exchanges oxygen and carbon dioxide between the air and the blood in the lungs. The nose filters, warms, and humidifies air before it travels through the pharynx (throat) through the glottis, the epiglottis, and vocal cords through the trachea and into the bronchi. The epiglottis prevents food from entering the larynx. The trachea is held open by C-shaped rings of cartilage to facilitate air flow. The bronchi (right and left) have cartilage to preserve the opening into the tertiary branches that open into the lung segments. Bronchioles connect each bronchial branch to alveoli (small elastic sacs where air is exchanged). The lungs contain the bronchial tree, bronchioles, and alveoli and each is surrounded by a pleural sac to facilitate movement. The diaphragm separates the lungs from the abdominal cavity. It contracts and moves downward to improve lung capacity for inspiration and relaxes and moves upward to facilitate exhalation.

Lymphatic system

The lymph system works to keep the body free from infections and at a stable temperature. The lymphatic capillaries in the gastrointestinal tract remove fat and transport it to the bloodstream. The lymph nodes filter lymph from all parts of the body and destroy infectious agents. The spleen filters out broken red blood cells. The thymus produces hormones during childhood and decreases in size as the body matures. It produces T lymphocytes in adults. Red bone marrow produces red and white blood cells. In response to injury, the lymphatic system produces histamine which causes swelling, capillary expansion and permeability. It calls WBCs to the site and produces pus from dead WBCs and bacteria. If the lymphatic system recognizes a foreign substance (antigen), it activates B and T cells to produce antibodies to attack the antigen. This system can develop active immunity that lasts a lifetime or passive immunity that is short-termed.

Nutrients

Nutrients are the substances the body uses for building, maintaining, and repairing. There are six kinds of nutrients: proteins for building; carbohydrates for energy, burning of fats for energy, and fiber to aid peristalsis; lipids (fats) for energy, insulation, and transportation of fat-soluble vitamins; vitamins for making body processes possible; minerals for controlling conservation and release of energy; and water for transportation of other nutrients, regulating body temperature, maintaining the chemical balance in the cells, removing waste, and lubricating joints. Without proper nutrition, the epithelium would deteriorate and the body would lose its protective barrier. The quality of nutrition determines the efficiency of repair of body tissues and the immune response to infectious attackers.

- *Protein:* Protein is made of essential and non-essential amino acids that form the building blocks for the body. Essential amino acids are those that must be obtained from the diet, and non-essential amino acids can be synthesized by the body if nitrogen is present. Complete proteins, found in animal products, supply the body with the materials necessary for building, repair, and growth. Incomplete proteins, found in plant sources, lack one or more amino acids. They do not aid growth, but they do provide for life. Deficient amounts of protein can cause crowded teeth or Kwashiorkor, which causes delayed eruption and hypoplasia. Proper protein consumption is important for the maintenance of healthy periodontal tissues and for fighting infectious diseases of the oral tissues.

- *Carbohydrates:* Carbohydrates are divided into simple or complex carbohydrates according to the number of monosaccharide molecules present. The monosaccharide glucose (blood sugar) is the form of carbohydrate most easily converted to energy by the body. Starch, the most nutritionally important carbohydrate, is derived from plants and is more slowly digested. Animal starch, called glycogen, is stored in the liver and regulates blood sugar, or in muscles to provide energy for muscle contraction. Dextran is the sugar used by *Streptococcus mutans* to produce dental caries. Fibers from plants are not digestible and pectin from fruit facilitates peristalsis. Various enzymes and hormones make digestion and absorption of carbohydrates possible. Insulin is the protein hormone produced by the pancreas to increase glucose absorption for energy.
- *Fats:* Like proteins and carbohydrates, fats are composed of carbon, hydrogen, and oxygen. They are divided into triglycerides (fats and oils), phospholipids, and sterols (cholesterol) (Nelson, 2000). About one tablespoon of essential fats is necessary for energy and insulation for the body. Fats carry fat-soluble nutrients and aid in absorption; they add flavor to foods; and they provide a feeling of appetite satisfaction. Saturated fats, with maximum hydrogen atoms, are found in animal fats and tropical oils. Monounsaturated fats, with ho hydrogen atoms, are derived from lamb, shortening, and olive and canola oils. They have no effect on serum cholesterol. Polyunsaturated fats, found in soybean, cottonseed, and vegetable oils, reduce serum cholesterol. Cholesterol comes from animal sources. Too much fat can produce plaque that adheres to the sides of the arteries and eventually closes them. Reduced fat diets and exercise are the principle deterrents to elevated serum cholesterol and blocked arteries.

- *Vitamins and minerals:* Vitamins and minerals do not provide energy to the body, but they allow the body to use the other nutrients to build, maintain, and repair. They help to regulate the release of energy. Fat-soluble vitamins are stored in the liver and fatty tissues and can become toxins if they are not used immediately. Water-soluble vitamins, such as the Bs and C, aid metabolism and the production and repair of body tissues. They are readily available in a well-balanced diet. Macro-minerals calcium and phosphorus and magnesium form the basis of bones and teeth and help to regulate cell metabolism. Magnesium, potassium, and chloride aid nerve functions. Sodium and chloride work to balance electrolytes, and all the macronutrients aid acid-base balance.

Function of water

Water makes up 50% to 60% of total body weight and resides in and around the cells; therefore it is essential for daily maintenance. Cell membranes are semi-permeable and allow water and other nutrients to flow in and out to maintain a balance between the cells and the bloodstream. Water is the medium for transporting nutrition to cells and wastes away from cells. It lubricates body parts, maintains body temperature, and reacts in chemical functions. Water is usually readily available. The body can dehydrate because of blood loss, vomiting or diarrhea, or because of insufficient intake. Survival without water is limited to about two days, possibly three days.

Microbiology, Immunology and Pharmacology

Bacterial concepts and classifications

Bacteria are the smallest living organisms that are a part of our daily lives. Some of them promote health while others cause health to deteriorate. Some bacteria live in peaceful co-existence with their hosts. Some bacteria must have oxygen to live; others can not live in the presence of oxygen. Still others adapt to the oxygen content of the environment in which they live. Bacteria have a binomial system; the Genus name is capitalized, and the species name is written in lower case letters. Both parts of the name are italicized. Bacteria are further classified according to their cell structure. Prokaryotes are unicellular and do not have a nucleus. Eukaryotes are more advanced and contain a nucleus and organelles. Viruses, helminths, and prions make up the remaining classifications of bacteria. Prions are the newly classified bacteria that are resistant to many forms of sterilization.

Observation of bacteria

Bacteria can be any size from one micrometer (μm = 10^{-6}) to a centimeter (cm = 10^{-2}). Living bacteria are usually viewed on a wet mount slide through a microscope. Acid/base stains show different cell components, and single dyes indicate polarization or lack of polarization characteristics. Bacteria have different shapes such as round (cocci) in pairs, chains, and four-square, eight-cube, and clusters. Bacilli are usually rods or cylinders; again they come in pairs, chains, with rounded ends, and with tapered ends. Spirella are spiral or a portion of a spiral. Bacteria can have a thick, organized coating or a slime layer. They can have flagella, filaments, pili, or fimbriae to aid attachment to cell walls and facilitate movement. The cell walls, plasma membrane, cell envelope, and internal structure work together to prevent cell death and to promote replication. Some gram-positive cells form spores in an undesirable environment to preserve life.

Bacterial growth

Bacteria grow when one parent divides into two. There are four distinct phases of bacterial growth; lag phase while they adjust to the environment, log phase in which they increase at logarithmic rates, stationary phase in which numbers are stable, and death phase when numbers decline. Colony-forming units (CFU) of bacteria and plaque-forming units (PFU) of viruses usually generate at about 20 minutes. Bacteria need proper temperature, pH, and good osmotic pressure to replicate. They require appropriate oxygen content and good nutrition to grow well. Three types of nutrition facilitate growth. Heterotrophic bacteria need organic compounds; autotrophic bacteria need inorganic compounds; and hypotrophic bacteria use whatever nutrition is available.

Destruction of bacteria

Bacteria can be destroyed chemically by inhibiting cell wall synthesis (penicillin and tetracycline), disrupting the cell membrane (polymycin), inhibiting DNA synthesis (rifampin), and by using drugs or chemicals that compete for nutrition (sulfa drugs). Mechanical sterilization also destroys bacteria. Antibiotics have become so widely used that drug-resistant bacteria have developed, and more research for stronger anti-bacterial chemicals is necessary. Sterilization (total destruction of all life forms, including spores) of dental instruments and disinfection (destruction of pathogenic organisms on hard surfaces) of objects which can not be sterilized are essential in the dental office. Weekly monitoring of sterilization efficacy and documentation of results are an important part of infection control.

Sterilization and disinfecting

Sterilization by various methods is critical for instruments that penetrate oral tissues. Steam (under pressure for 15 – 20 minutes at 250 - 270° F at 15 – 20 lbs of pressure) causes coagulation of protein and death for all life forms, including spores. Dry heat for one hour at 320 - 350° F causes oxidation of cell parts. Unsaturated chemical vapor for 20 – 30 minutes at 270° F at the pressure set by manufacturers is especially good for orthodontic wires, but the vapors are toxic. Ethylene oxide at 120° F for 2 – 3 hours or at room temperature for 8 – 10 hours destroys bacteria; it, too, has toxic vapors. Immersion in glutaraldehyde chloride dioxide is the best sterilization solution for heat sensitive instruments, but monitoring of efficacy is not possible. Weekly spore tests that use a control added to the pack is the best way to monitor the efficacy of sterilization methods.

High level disinfectants inactivate bacteria, including spores, fungi, and viruses, and can be classified as sterilization solutions if the items are immersed for the proper length of time. This category includes bleach (in 1:10 solution, mixed daily) and iodophors (mixed daily). Intermediate level disinfectants such as chlorhexidine, inactivate many microorganisms and low level disinfectants inactivate vegetative bacteria and some viruses. Iodophors and chlorhexidine have residual action. Every disinfectant used in the dental office should have EPA approval as tuberculocidal, bacteriocidal, virucidal, and fungicidal with adequate instructions for shelf life and use life. Alcohols are effective skin cleansers and to pre-clean instruments. Hydrogen peroxide rinse is effective for debriding wounds and destroying anaerobic bacteria. Soaps are effective only as wetting agents.

Human immune response

The body has nonspecific defenses against disease as well as defenses designed to protect from specific microorganisms. Some defensive bacteria live in the mouth, the digestive tract and on the skin. Physical barriers such as skin, mucous membranes, and body fluids work with white blood cells and the lymph system to protect, and inflammation surrounds and damages non-specific foreign substances when necessary. Specific immunity comes through exposure to the particular disease, immunity through fetal blood circulation, or by injection of a serum. T-lymphocytes respond to altered cell surfaces and produce delayed hypersensitivity (Type IV). Sometimes the body exaggerates the immune response causing an allergic response. Occasionally the immune response is not effective due to the use of prescription drugs, or the body actually attacks itself.

Types of infections

Gingivitis and periodontitis are the principle diseases of the oral cavity. Plaque made from waste products of digestion and oral flora adheres to the teeth attracting more minerals from saliva. If salivary flow is sufficient, it can increase the pH above 5.5 to reduce the growth of caries-causing bacteria. However, insufficient salivary flow can allow the teeth to be bathed in acidic saliva for 20 to 120 minutes after eating. Without adequate plaque removal the bacteria travels toward the apical surface of teeth, deepening the sulcus and changing from aerobic gram-positive bacteria to anaerobic gram-negative bacteria. At this point the gingiva begins to exhibit signs of inflammation. Further neglect allows the bacteria to begin destruction of periodontal ligaments and eventually bone.

Gingivitis is reversible when the patient begins proper oral hygiene and/or hormones stabilize. Neglected gingivitis continues to destroy periodontal structures, becomes periodontitis, and eventually causes tooth loss. Medical research is now connecting low birth weight babies as well as heart disease and increased problems with diabetes to poor oral hygiene and periodontitis. Aggressive periodontitis (formerly known as juvenile periodontitis) seems to have more to do with genetics than with oral hygiene, and it can affect primary teeth. It causes rapid loss of alveolar bone. Necrotizing periodontal disease (ANUG) causes cratering of interdental papilla, rapid destruction of PDL and bone. It can occur as a result of stress as well as compromised immunity.

Infections of epithelial tissues

Dental health care workers are subject to infections of epithelial tissues such as herpes simplex, varicella zoster (chicken pox and shingles), measles, rubella, and mumps through respiratory droplets and mononucleosis through direct contact with saliva. Bacterial infections such as tetnus, *Staphylococcus aureus, Streptococcus pyogenes,* and *Pseudomonas aeruginosa,* and fungal infections such as candidiasis can enter through cuts or wounds or with inhalation of respiratory droplets. Thorough review of the medical history with the patient alerts the health care worker to the presence of these infections before the oral examination begins. In addition, wearing proper personal protection equipment and using adequate infection control measures prevent cross-contamination with the patient.

Respiratory infections

Colds are caused by a virus and are usually self-limiting. Strep throat is another common respiratory problem that patients deliver to health care workers. However, strep throat usually needs to be treated with antibiotics. Diphtheria, a more serious respiratory infection spread by respiratory droplets must be treated by a primary care physician. Whooping cough (pertussis) causes convulsive coughing. Pneumonia and influenza are highly contagious if the patient has a fever. There are vaccines available for each of these except colds and strep throat; however, the health care worker should avoid exposure whenever possible. The dental health care worker is less likely to have a patient with legionnaire's disease or cytomegalovirus unless the disease is in the early stage before diagnosis.

Gastrointestinal infections

Hepatitis in its various forms was the best known and most feared viral disease for health care workers until HIV (human immunodeficiency virus) became widely known. Hepatitis A and E are transmitted most often by oral-fecal routes such as contaminated water and food sources and inadequate sewage disposal. Hepatitis B, C, D, and G are spread through blood and plasma products, sexual transmission, or through contaminated needles. Each of these forms of hepatitis can also be transmitted from a mother to her child at birth. Hepatitis D is found only in conjunction with HBV, and hepatitis G is a co-infection with hepatitis C. Vaccines are available for HAV and HBV, and infection control measures equal to those set out by the CDC, thorough hand-washing and proper sanitation are the best defenses against other hepatitis forms. Bacterial food poisoning (*Clostridium botulinum* and *Staphylococcus aureus)* is usually transmitted through contaminated food.

Potential infections for dental workers

Infective endocarditis is significant to dental health care workers because possible damage to heart valves can leave him/her susceptible to further endocarditis. Staph or strep bacteria can enter the health care worker's blood stream through a cut or deep scratch and cause the same damage as in other situations.

Haemophilus meningitis and poliomyelitis are spread mainly through inhalation of respiratory droplets; there are vaccines available. Conjunctivitis (pink eye) can be caused by one of several viruses, but each can cause scarring and blindness if the droplets of exudates spread into the DHCW eyes. The health care worker's best defense is a thorough medical history and extra-oral exam while wearing safety glasses and gloves.

Dental office drug use

Several drugs are used in the dental office as analgesics to relieve pain during treatment and post-operatively. Anesthetics should be chosen with care to prevent a respiratory or cardiac crisis. Some patients need medications before the dental treatment to relieve anxiety. And many patients need short-term, light sedation during treatment. Occasionally, the patient needs an antibiotic to reduce bacterial infection before treatment can begin. The dental health care worker must review and update the patient's health history with the patient each time the patient is in the office for treatment. He/she should notice any changes in history or medications to prevent inadvertently using or prescribing a drug that will interact negatively with current health problems or medications.

Analgesics

Analgesics generally work to desensitize the nerve endings and dull the patient's perception of discomfort or pain. Salicylates (aspirin) and nonsteroidal anti-inflammatory agents (NSAIAs/NSAIDs) work well to reduce mild to moderate pain, and to decrease fever and inflammation. They irritate the GI tract and can cause bleeding due to their ability to inhibit platelet clotting. Aspirin can interact with warfarin to decrease blood clotting even more, and with many antihypertensive medications to diminish their efficacy. Acetaminophen reduces pain and fever, but it can cause liver and kidney toxicity with long-term use. Opioid analgesics and antagonists relieve moderate to severe pain depending on the dosage. They decrease coughing as well as providing analgesia. They can also cause nausea and vomiting and constipation. Respiratory difficulties, restlessness, and anxiety are also common adverse reactions.

Anti-infectives

Anti-infective agents work "against or destroy infections". These agents can be bactericidal (kill bacteria), bacteriostatic (inhibit or retard bacterial growth), antibiotic (produced by another microorganism to kill or inhibit growth), antimicrobial, or antiviral. The efficacy of an anti-infective agent depends on the concentration of the agent in the blood, resistance by the invading microorganism, the polarity of the drug (gram-positive or gram-negative) and the immune response of the host. A drug that has too low concentration in the host blood, or is not designed for the invading microorganism can cause drug resistance by the microorganism. If one anti-infective drug is used without complete success and another drug is prescribed, care should be taken that the two drugs are compatible and complimentary so that both are effective.

Specific anti-infective mechanisms

Penicillins work best against gram-positive bacteria, but are effective against some gram-negative cocci. Penicillinase is reserved for use only against penicillinase-producing staphylococci. Amoxicillin has an extended spectrum against both gram-positive and gram-negative bacteria, but does not work well against penicillinase-resistant bacteria. Macrolides (erythromycin, azithromycin, and clarithromycin) have some activity against anaerobes. Tetracyclines cause intrinsic staining of permanent teeth if given to children before about nine years of age. Clindamycin is good for oral and bone infections and for endocarditis prophylaxis. Penicillins, macrolides, tetracyclines, clindamycin, cephalosporins, and aminoglycosides inhibit or prevent cell wall or protein synthesis. Metronidazole (Flagyl) is trichomonacidal as well as bactericidal. Sulfonamides compete for receptor sites, and quinolones inhibit nucleic acid and synthesis. Antifungal agents are prescribed for skin or mucosal lesions. Antiviral agents prescribed are for herpes simplex viruses, and anti-tuberculosis agents are reserved for use by primary care physicians or pulmonary specialists.

Local anesthetics

Local anesthetics prevent nerves from carrying sensation away from the nerve membrane at the injection site. The anesthetic, being basic (pH less than 7.4) penetrates the tissue easily in its ionized form. However, inflamed tissue, being more acidic, slows penetration and potency of the anesthetic. The local nerve loses it function first at the autonomic level, then cold sensation, then warmth, pain, touch, pressure, vibration, proprioception, and finally motor response. Sensation returns in reverse order. The drug, its concentration, route of administration, rate of injection, vascularity, patient's weight, and rate of metabolism, and excretion effect toxicity. Most local anesthetics contain a vasoconstrictor to reduce systemic toxicity, an antioxidant to stabilize the solution in the carpule, an alkalinizing agent to keep the pH between six and seven, and sodium chloride to make the solution isotonic.

Anti-anxiety drugs

Sedatives are mild CNS depressants that make the patient more calm. Hypnotics are stronger and will cause the patient to sleep. Minor tranquilizers work very much like sedatives and hypnotics, but major tranquilizers are used to decrease psychotic activity. Benzodiazepines (Valium and Ativan) are easily absorbed and metabolized. The strength of the dose determines the depth of CNS depression. Buspirone (Buspar) is not used for dental anxiety. Barbiturates (Pentothal, Seconal, and Luminal) cause CNS depression for light sedation to respiratory and cardiovascular arrest depending on the dose. They are contraindicated for people with a family history of porphyria. Possible acute poisoning and many drug interactions must be considered before prescribing barbiturates. Non-barbiturate sedative hypnotic drugs (Noctec, Equanil, and Miltown) are used for preoperative sedation for children, but are not for adults. Centrally acting muscle relaxants affect the CNS and are prescribed for muscle spasms.

General anesthetics

General anesthetics are potent CNS depressants which cause reversible loss of consciousness and insensitivity to pain. There are four stages of anesthesia:

- *I – Analgesia*
- *II – Delirium or excitement (done quickly)*
- *III – Surgical anesthesia:* Four planes, in which most treatment is performed
- *IV – Respiratory paralysis:* This must be reversed quickly or the patient will die. Stage IV is not purposely used. Inhalation anesthetics provide relaxation and quick induction and recovery.

N2O is safe for children and provides analgesia and amnesia. Halogenated hydrocarbons are unpopular because of possible occurrence of post-anesthetic hepatitis. Halogenated ether is useful and popular. Ultra short-acting barbiturates (Brevital and Pentothal IV) are used for rapid transition to Stage III. They can cause laryngospasm and bronchospasm, and are contraindicated for patients with status asthmaticus, porphyria, and hypersensitivity. Ketamine (IV or IM) can cause delirium and hallucinations during recovery. Opiates are useful for pre-anesthesia and analgesia. Benzodiazepine helps with induction of anesthesia.

Emergency drugs

Emergency drugs vary in the dental office according to preference of the ACLS-trained personnel. Epinephrine is used for cardiac stimulation, vasoconstriction, bronchial dilation, and elevation of blood glucose. Benadryl is an antihistamine used to reduce allergic reactions. Valium is used for most convulsions if a drug is needed; it produces toxic reaction to local anesthetic. Narcan is given for Opioid-induced apnea. Oxygen returns proper 02 saturation to hemoglobin. Aromatic ammonia spirits stimulates respiratory action. Glucose restores balance of blood glucose. Morphine relieves pain and reduces apprehension of cardiac infarction. Methoxamine slightly increases blood pressure. Nitroglycerin relaxes heart muscle and reduces its work. Hydrocortisone is needed for allergic reactions, anaphylaxis, and adrenal crisis. Dextrose (IV) manages an unconscious diabetic patient. Metaproterenol relieves broncho-constriction.

Cardiovascular disease or seizure disorders

Hypertension, angina, stroke, atherosclerosis, and congestive heart failure in addition to myocardial infractions and surgeries affect dental treatment. Each problem carries specific medications to reduce or correct the problem. A review of an updated medical history with the patient is essential before dental treatment is started. The dental health care worker should notice medications that increase cardiac production or improve rhythms and guard against recommending a contraindicated medicine. Anti-hypertensives, anti-coagulants, and anti-hyperlipidemics in the medical history are reminders to monitor vital signs.

Patients with one of two types of seizure disorders are commonly seen in the dental office. The absence *(petit mal)* seizure patient loses consciousness, but has no muscular reaction. The patient with tonic-clonic *(grand mal)* seizures presents jerking muscular movements and should be prevented from harming him/herself until EMT help arrives. Detailed medical history, control of medication side effects and stress management are important issues with this patient.

Psychiatric disorders

Patients with schizophrenia have trouble determining reality. The phenothiazine drugs normally prescribed calm the emotions, but they also can produce Parkinsonism, orthostatic hypotension, xerostomia, blurred vision, and blood dyscrasias. They also decrease the efficacy of opioids and increase the effects of anticholinergic agents. First generation (tricyclic) antidepressants can cause tremors, sedation, xerostomia, orthostatic hypotension, myocardial toxicity and interactions with other drugs and some foods. Second generation antidepressants have many of the same adverse effects of tricyclics. Lithium, used for anxiety, phobia, bipolar disorder and obsessive-compulsive disorder can cause problems with NSAIDs as well as other drugs. All these drugs present problems with drug interactions, manual dexterity, and orthostatic hypotension.

Dental treatment and hormones

Adrenal glands secrete glucocorticoids; cortisol (hydrocortisone) is response to stress (fight or flight). Hydrocortisone inhibits the release of ACTH and suppresses inflammation and allergic reactions. Adverse reactions are relative to length of therapy and dosage, and include increased or masked infection, personality or behavior changes, peptic ulcer, ineffective wound healing, and osteoporosis. Hydrocortisone treats asthma and autoimmune diseases such as arthritis; therefore, dosage might need adjusting for dental treatment.

Pituitary hormone treats diabetes insipidus and clotting disorders. Thyroid hormone effects physiological function. CNS depressants must be used with caution when the patient has hypothyroidism. If the patient has hyperthyroidism, epinephrine is contraindicated and the appointment must lack stress. The pancreatic hormones, glucagons and insulin, are produced in the islets of Langerhans. The diabetic patient may have periodontal disease due to inadequate circulation and immune response. Female and male hormones affect dental treatment only if the patient is taking anabolic steroids to build muscle mass.

Allergic reactions

Autacoid is the natural host response to allergic reaction; antihistamine blocks histamine receptors and reduces allergic reaction. Prostaglandin, thromboxanes, leukotrienes, and kinins are produced in response to inflammation or injury. They increase body temperature and capillary permeability. They also are part of the periodontal inflammation and alveolar bone resorption process.

Asthma is an allergic response. Mucus collects, airways are restricted, and expiratory airflow is decreased. Drugs reduce the allergic reaction and open bronchial airways. COPD –chronic obstructive pulmonary disease – is the irreversible result of chronic bronchitis and/or emphysema. N2O causes hypoxia in the COPD patient. Other respiratory therapy drugs cause dry mouth, adrenergic stimulation, candidiasis, and reduced immune response to infections. Stress reduction and chair positioning to reduce airway obstruction are indicated in addition to elimination of drug interactions and physician consultations.

GI disease and/or chemotherapy

Patients with gastrointestinal disorders take medications designed to neutralize acids or prevent the release of acids or to promote peristalsis. Care should be taken to prevent interaction between any of those medications and medications prescribed for dental treatment. Finding appointment times that are comfortable for the patient and managing the side effects of sedation, dizziness, and dry mouth relieve some of the patient's discomfort.

Chemotherapeutic agents designed to destroy malignant cells also reduce the efficacy of the natural immunity of the patient. Working in conjunction with the oncologist to eliminate dental disease before chemotherapy, then providing alcohol-free fluoride products and palliative oral rinses provide the patient's best chance for preserving dental health during chemotherapy.

Benign and malignant neoplasms

Neoplasms grow slowly or rapidly, but growth of abnormal cells is uncontrolled. They originate from viral or chemical sources or from exposure to radiation. Ameloblastomas, epithelial tumors related to enamel cells, papillomas, and salivary gland pleomorphic adenoma should be removed.

Benign neoplasms have cellular structure that closely resembles the structure of normal tissue nearby. They are usually encapsulated. Benign neoplasms are significant because they may interfere with proper function of nearby organs. Soft tissue neoplasms such as fibromas, like vascular neoplasms such as hemangiomas and melanocytic nevi, are usually benign, but removal and biopsy are sometimes necessary.

Malignant neoplasms present rapidly replicating cell structure that can spread into nearby tissues. These are most often found in lungs, digestive organs, and sex organs. Kaposi's sarcoma, malignant melanoma, and osteosarcoma are malignant. They, like squamous cell carcinoma, basal cell carcinoma, adenoid cystic carcinoma, and mucoepidermoid carcinoma must be surgically removed.

Blood disorders

Red blood cell disorders include anemias and polycythemias. Anemias occur when the concentration of hemoglobin and oxygen in the blood gets too low. Anemia can be caused by bleeding, hemolysis, iron or other nutrient deficiency, or improper formation of new red blood cells. Polycythemias are caused by too many red blood cells with too little oxygen in the blood.

Hemophilia is a genetic disease in which blood does not have the proper proteins to make it clot. Treatment includes blood transfusions and/or placing clotting proteins in the blood before dental/hygiene treatment.

White blood cell diseases of leukocytes and bone marrow include leukemia (cancer of red bone marrow or lymphatic tissue) and agranulocytosis (a severe lack of basophils, eosinophils, or neutrophils). Exact causes for leukemia are not known, but research indicates that genetics, radiation and/or viruses could be causes. Agranulocytosis may be caused by immune system malfunction, medications, or radiation.

Skin disorders

Dermatitis refers to acute or chronic inflammation of the skin. Eczema presents non-specific lesions and itching. Seborrheic dermatitis involves redness, inflammation of sebaceous glands, itching, and scaling. Psoriasis patients have raised papules of patches with silvery scales and thickened skin on extremities. Infectious skin diseases can be caused by bacteria or viruses. Acne, multiple facial lesions caused by plugged sebaceous glands, can be triggered by hormones, stress, or drugs. Abscesses, also called boils or furuncles, look like raised pockets of necrotic tissue with purulent exudate; they are usually around trauma sites or obstructed skin appendages. Localized viral infections, such as warts, are a proliferation of squamous epithelium and may disappear spontaneously.

Metabolic disorders

Overproduction is usually caused by a tumor in the gland, and hypo-secretion occurs because the secretory cells are blocked or destroyed. The pituitary overproduction of growth hormone causes giantism and acromegaly. Hypo-function causes diabetes insipidus. Too much thyroxine causes tachycardia, weight loss, and protruding eyes of Graves' disease. Hypo-thyroidism causes dwarfism and underdevelopment. If the adrenal gland overproduces, the patient presents obesity, easy bruising, hyperglycemia, and hypertension. Under production causes dehydration, unbalanced electrolytes, low blood pressure, and weight loss. Liver diseases can cause destruction of the liver with fibrous regeneration. Viral hepatitis affects about 2 of 1,000 persons in the US each year. Patients present anorexia, malaise, jaundice, and enlarged liver.

Diabetes mellitus and pancreatitis occur when the pancreas malfunctions. Diabetes mellitus results from inadequate insulin or inadequate response to insulin. Pancreatitis is caused by protein and lipid-digesting enzymes digesting the pancreas.

Pathology

"Pathology is the study of the destruction and repair of bodily tissues". Injury can be caused by chemical, physical, or microbial agents, immunological response, nutritional deficiencies, or genetics. The body responds to injury or attack by generating inflammation. Acute inflammation causes blood flow to increase, blood vessels to become more permeable, and leukocytes, primarily neutrophils, to rush to clean up necrotic debris and destroy, neutralize, or remove the attacker. Chronic inflammation is the body's response to a long-lasting injury and repair that occur at the same time. That "inflammatory response" regenerates injured cells by replacing them with cells of the same type. Repair is the restoring of cell function by adding connective tissue through angiogenesis, remodeling, and fibrosis.

Oral Pathology and History

Variant oral conditions

Some oral conditions that are considered variations of normal include:

- Fordyce granules are asymptomatic clusters of yellow lobules of sebaceous origin.
- Tori are extra bone found on the central palate or bilaterally on the mandible in the cuspid to first molar area.
- Pigmentation can exhibit differences in color (usually darker) on the mucosa.
- Linea alba is a white line at the occlusal plane on the buccal mucosa.
- Leukoedema is a generalized white film located bilaterally on the buccal mucosa and is caused by edema in the buccal spinous cells.
- Lingual thyroid nodule presents a small, nodular mass slightly behind the circumvallate papillae.
- Fissured tongue looks like deep grooves on top of the tongue.
- Geographic tongue is patchy area of the tongue from which the filiform papillae are gone and is usually caused by stress, heredity, or nutrition.
- Hairy tongue, usually caused by antibiotics, shows overgrown areas of filiform papillae.
- Lingual varices are enlarged veins or arteries on the ventral surface of the tongue.

Placing dental implants

Evaluation of the patient's oral hygiene, medical and dental history, motivation for success of implant, and the amount of bone present are all necessary planning steps when considering placement of dental implants. Adequate ability to heal is important, but motivation to continue excellent oral hygiene is essential. The patient's motivation to keep all evaluation appointments before the final crown is placed is equally important. Evaluations between implant placement and final crown placement provide opportunities to assess healing and integration. Dental implants can fail because of infection or because the bone and implant did not integrate properly. The implant can become mobile, and radiographs show decreased bone support and radiolucency around the implant. Early intervention by debridement and immaculate oral hygiene can sometimes revive the implant before it fails completely.

Oral hyperplasias

A pyogenic granuloma, found on lips, tongue, or buccal mucosa, can be caused by hormonal changes or chronic irritants. It is similar to giant cell granuloma, and usually can be differentiated only by a biopsy. A removable prosthesis can cause fibrous projections or hyperplastic folds of tissue near the edge of the prosthesis. Gingival hyperplasias can be caused by irritants, hormones, and poor oral hygiene. Sometimes fibromas develop in response to irritants and must be surgically removed. Ulcerations can be the result of trauma or, in the case of aphthous ulcers, emotional stress. Aphthous ulcers, also known as canker sores, found on unattached mucosa are usually small (≤ 1 cm) single lesions. A herpetiform aphthous ulcer has small clusters of lesions. Traumatic ulcers can result from biting, irritation from a prosthesis, or trauma from food. Like canker sores, these usually last from 7 – 14 days and need only palliative treatment.

Etiology of periapical lesions

An abscess causing pain, sometimes exudate, and radiological changes, can develop in the pulp or periapical tissues. It can be the result of trauma or a bacterial infection, and is usually resolved by endodontic treatment or extraction of the involved tooth. Cementomas are lesions caused by disordered cementum and bone. The tooth is vital and asymptomatic. Radicular cysts are lined with epithelium and are differentiated from periapical granulomas by biopsy. Periapical granulomas involve chronic growth of granulation tissue and are resolved by endodontic treatment or tooth extraction. Condensing osteitis is an asymptomatic response to an infection in the bone around a tooth (frequently first molar) that looks more radiopaque around the tooth. Alveolar osteitis (dry socket) results when the blood clot in an extraction site is improperly formed or lost. Chronic hyperplastic pulpitis is an asymptomatic polyp in the middle of a large carious lesion.

Immunologic disorders

Three categories of immunological disorders:

- Hypersensitivity responses can be mild or anaphylactic. Simply avoiding the irritant can resolve minor cases, or epinephrine, oxygen, and medical assistance may be needed.
- Pathogenic lesions resembling targets are called erythema multiforme. They are red macules and ulcerations on the mucosa or tongue. The most severe form is called Stevens-Johnson syndrome. Corticosteriods remedy these lesions.
- Lichen planus is benign, chronic and has one of four forms – atrophic, erosive, reticular (thin white lines called Wickham's striae and white papules), or plaque-like. The epithelial layer separates from the connective tissue in the erosive and bulbous form. Treatment is palliative.

- Lupus erythematosus is chronic and progressively affects skin and organs. A butterfly rash over the bridge of the nose is classic sign. It is treated with steroids or aspirin.
- Pemphigus vulgaris and benign mucous membrane pemphigoid affect skin and cause separation of epithelium and connective tissue. It is treated with corticoids.

Odontogenic cysts

A *dentigerous cyst,* sometimes called a *follicular cyst*, is caused by disturbed enamel epithelium, and forms around an unerupted tooth. This is treated by removing the cyst and the tooth. An *eruption cyst* is soft tissue swelling around a newly erupted crown, and resolves itself as the tooth erupts. A *primordial cyst* develops where a tooth should be, and is caused by disturbed enamel organ. It is well-defined, unilocular or multilocular, and usually in the third molar area. Removal is necessary. An *odontogenic keratocyst* is lined with epithelium and parakeratin; it can move and/or resorb teeth. It is well-defined, multilocular, and radiolucent, and most often in the third molar area. Treatment is excision, but the cyst can return. A *lateral periodontal cyst* is asymptomatic in soft tissue or bone and indicated by swollen interdental papillae. It is found most often in mandibular cuspid or premolar area and must be removed.

Non-odontogenic cysts

Nasopalatine, median palatine, globulomaxillary, and nasolabial cysts are named for their locations. All are radiolucent. These are usually asymptomatic, and each is treated by excision. Epidermoid cysts involve epithelium cells, and dermoid cysts involve epithelium, mesoderm, and endoderm. These are in the mandible and require removal. Static bone cyst, in the lingual mandibular bone concavity, has no epithelial lining. It is caused by a depression in the side of the mandible where part of the salivary gland is located. It requires no treatment. Simple bone cyst (traumatic bone cyst) is a well-defined radiolucency found frequently between mandibular molar roots. Aneurysmal bone cyst look like a soap bubble on radiographs, and may cause bone expansion. Both simple bone cysts and aneurysmal bone cysts must be removed.

Medical and dental history

Patient history

The social history includes personal demographic information about the patient. It provides information necessary to set appointments, legal permission for treatment, and acknowledgement that the patient has received HIPPA information. The patient's attitude toward the importance of dental care for a healthy mouth is a significant part of the social history.

The health history provides information about current medications, allergies, conditions being treated by physicians, current diseases and conditions, and any conditions that might affect dental treatment. Dental health history provides information regarding oral hygiene and personal habits such as nail biting, grinding teeth during sleep, and clenching or grinding teeth in times of stress.

Vital signs – blood pressure, body temperature, pulse, and respirations - provide the health care worker with information about the patient at the time of the appointment

Pre-visit information

Time is the major impediment to acquiring sufficient information to begin dental treatment during a telephone interview. The receptionist can remind the patient to bring a list of health problems and medications to the initial appointment along with insurance information. A questionnaire completed by the patient gives the patient more time to consider his/her health history and to list current medications. The patient usually hurries through this task and forgets some information. An interview provides time for the health care worker and patient to build a bond that helps the patient to feel comfortable. However an interview, alone, is very time-consuming. An interview combined with a questionnaire allows the health care worker to learn more information about specific items on the health history, and it allows more time for the patient to remember relevant information.

Past illnesses and current medications

Past illnesses affect conditions presented by the patient, and past experiences affect current attitudes of the patient. Hypertension and the medications necessary to control it cause the patient to present tachycardia if he/she hurries to keep his/her appointment on time. Local anesthetics containing epinephrine are contra-indicated for the patient with hypertension because epinephrine speeds up the heart beat. Appointing after a meal and having a sugar source easily accessible is important for diabetic patients. Patients who have a seizure disorder must have a calm, non-eventful appointment to prevent another seizure. Patients who have a history of corrective heart surgery or bacterial endocarditis are very susceptible to bacterial endocarditis and must be premedicated with an antibiotic an hour before dental treatment. Each health problem presents particular treatment considerations to prevent occurrence or recurrence of a health episode.

Blood pressure

Blood pressure, average for adults is 120/80 mm Hg, is the force against the walls of the arteries when the heart pumps blood. Sphygmomanometer is the flexible cuff that fits around the patient's upper arm, the bulb with which the cuff is inflated, and the manometer or device that indicates the pressure. The proper size of cuff should be about 20% bigger than the diameter of the arm. A cuff that is too small will provide a higher reading than is correct, and a cuff that is too large will provide an incorrect reading that is lower than it actually is. The most accurate sphygmomanometer is the mercury column. The stethoscope, consisting of earpieces, binaurals (connects earpieces to tubing), the tubing from the binaurals to the chest piece, and chest piece, amplifies the sound and allows the health care worker to hear the heart sounds.

Thermometers

Patient's temperature can be measured with a disposable (single use) thermometer which eliminates cross-contamination, a mercury in a glass tube thermometer (must be sanitized after each use), an electronic thermometer which gives digital readout, is very time efficient, and decreases cross-contamination, or a tympanic thermometer which is placed in the patient's ear and measures infrared energy emitted from the eardrum. The normal temperature range for adults is between 98.6°F and 100.6°F, and the normal temperature for children is 96.6°F to 100.6°F. Temperatures can vary with the time of day as well as a response to exercise, dehydration, or illness. Starvation, hemorrhage, and physiological shock can cause body temperature to decrease.

Pulse and respirations

The pulse is an indirect measurement of the rhythms and production of the heart and respirations indicate the body's efficacy at providing oxygen to peripheral tissues. The health care worker measures and/or monitors the patient's pulse to determine the immediate status of the patient's cardiac health. The HCW can palpate for the pulse at several arteries – radial, brachial, facial, temporal, or carotid; however the most easily accessible pulse is found at the radial artery. The HCW places two fingers on the patient's wrist at the radial artery and counts the number, rhythm, and strength of the pulse. Normal rate for adults is 60 – 80 beats per minute and for children is 90 – 120 beats per minute.

Measuring respirations provides the HCW with the immediate status of the patient's oxygen supply. Patients who present with a history of respiratory problems may need consideration for the placement of the chair, or the use or non-use of nitrous oxide sedation. Normal respirations are usually about 14 – 20 respirations and exhalations per minute.

Dental health history

Knowing the patient's history helps the dental health care worker to plan how to care for that patient best. For example, if the DHCW knows that the patient had a traumatic dental experience as a child or as an adult, the DHCW also knows that the patient is probably uncomfortable in the chair. This patient probably should have short appointments, and possibly needs nitrous oxide during the appointment. Occasionally, this type patient needs premedication and someone to drive him/her to and from the appointment. Patients with a history of periodontal disease frequently need three or four maintenance appointments each year with thorough periodontal evaluation at each appointment. Patients with multiple restorations need those restorations carefully monitored to prevent recurrent problems.

Patients with systemic challenges frequently need special care as dental patients. A patient with epilepsy usually takes an antispasmodic medication that causes gingival hyperplasia, tenderness and excessive bleeding. That patient needs specific oral rinses to reduce general bacterial flora in the mouth and continuing encouragement at follow-up appointments. After good oral hygiene is established, the patient may need gingival surgery if the hyperplasia interferes with brushing and flossing, or he may need more frequent appointments to reduce the risk for periodontal disease. Patients with diabetes may need frequent appointments to control the risk for periodontal disease since diabetic patients usually have slow healing times. Patients with physical handicaps may need special hygiene aids that are easier to hold. Generally, anything that affects the patient's health affects dental health as well.

During the review of the questionnaire filled out by the patient, the dental health care worker should ask if there are any current problems with dental health. A brief documentation of the complaint, length of time the problem has existed, and the extent of the discomfort alerts the dentist to the problem. History of past dental problems informs the dentist of whether the complaint is chronic or new. The dental history should also include any care provided by specialists such as orthodontists, periodontists, and/or TMJ specialists. Documentation should be made regarding oral hygiene habits and the number of times the patient visits the hygienist for dental prophylaxis and gingival treatments each year. The patient's attitude toward oral hygiene at home and at the dental office should also be written in the record.

Head and neck examination

Extra-oral examination

The extra-oral exam provides information regarding the overall look of the patient outside the oral cavity. The symmetry of the patient's face and the presence of swelling or lesions of systemic disease are readily apparent. Palpation, either bilaterally or bimanually, gives further information of asymmetrical structures or tissues of the head and neck. Listening in addition to palpation can inform the health care worker of TMJ crepitation. Palpation of the lymph nodes indicates the presence or absence of inflammation or an infection in the area of the head superior to those nodes. Observing whether the patient breathes through his/her mouth or nose supplies information about a deviated septum or swollen nasal passages. Listening to the patient's breathing gives clues to a possible stuffy nose or respiratory infection. The dental health care worker must be aware of the patient's general health in order to provide the best dental care.

Cracked and swollen lips

The hygienist should be concerned with a patient's cracked or swollen lips and for ulcerated lesions on the buccal mucosa. The first reason for concern by the hygienist should be the patient's discomfort associated with these conditions and the reduced level of good oral hygiene attending these conditions. Second reason for concern is whether the patient is presenting signs of an infectious disease that can be communicated to other patients or dental staff. Next, the hygienist is concerned because he/she knows that a patient with this level of discomfort can not tolerate the manipulation necessary for a thorough examination and dental prophylaxis treatment. Finally, and not as important as the other considerations, is the consideration of the productive time lost by the hygienist and the dental practice when a patient arrives for dental prophylaxis treatment with conditions that contraindicate treatment.

Palpating glands

The hygienist should palpate the sublingual gland and the parotid gland and the duct during the head and neck examination. The sublingual gland, located under the tongue, provides saliva to keep mucosa moist and to facilitate food digestion. The parotid gland is a major gland located in the upper cheek area under the cheek bone. It supplies saliva to clean the maxillary molars and to facilitate digestion of food. Palpating the gland and the duct (called milking) expresses saliva into the mouth and indicates proper functioning. A swollen parotid gland could indicate a virus infection. A lump in the gland or a blockage in the duct could indicate a tumor, or less seriously, a saliva stone. Saliva in the area would be reduced, food would be trapped, and bacteria would multiply causing gingival swelling, loss of periodontal integrity, decay and possible loss of those teeth.

Examining lymph nodes

The lymph nodes in the head and neck provide drainage for tissues and filtration for fluids in the head and neck. Painful, swollen, or fixed lymph nodes generally indicate an infection in the tissues superior to those nodes. Occasionally the patient remembers having a cold or respiratory infection that is waning, but sometimes a swollen or fixed lymph node alerts the patient and health care worker of a more serious problem. All of the lymph nodes are examined for pain, swelling, enlargement, and unusual hardness. The occipital lymph nodes are palpated bilaterally with the patient's head tilted forward. Auricular and parotid lymph nodes are examined by bilateral palpation. With the patient's head to the side, the hygienist uses his/her fingers to palpate the superficial cervical lymph nodes from anterior to posterior to the sternocleidomastoid muscle. The deep cervical lymph nodes are examined with the patient's head upright while the hygienist palpates along the sternocleidomastoid muscles with the thumb and fingers.

Lesion on nose

The patient presents with a crusty lesion on his nose. Usually the first question is to learn what caused the lesion. Is it because of a scratch or was it originally a small, elevated papule? The hygienist should learn if the lesion has healed and returned and how long the lesion has been there. Does the patient have a history of being exposed to the sun? The answers to these questions determine whether there should be further examination and perhaps a biopsy to learn if the lesion is cancerous. Basal cell carcinoma frequently begins as a small, elevated papule in the middle third of the face which heals, returns, crusts over, and repeats the sequence. The thought that healing occurs is deceptive because the lesion, if it is cancerous, spreads under the skin and into deeper tissue. A small scratch that happened recently would be insignificant.

Temporomandibular joint dysfunction

Temporomandibular joint dysfunction can cause chronic pain when the patient talks, chews his/her food, and clenches or grinds his/her teeth during sleep. The patient may talk about non-specific jaw pain or very specific pain in the area of the joint. Occasionally the patient tells about the jaw "locking" open or closed. TMJ dysfunction can also cause uneven wear facets on the teeth which can lead to further damage and the need for restoration. The patient's subjective observations should be noted and a physical exam performed. The hygienist should palpate bilaterally with index fingers in front of the ear. As the patient opens and closes his/her mouth, the hygienist listens for popping or clicking and observes deviations or restricted opening.

Periodontal evaluation

Reasons for evaluation

The periodontium, including gingiva, periodontal ligaments and bone, is the foundation for holding the teeth. Most periodontal problems are slow in developing, but juvenile periodontitis has rapid onset and destruction of periodontal tissues. Adults can have systemic problems that first show up in the periodontal tissues. And, anyone with a history of periodontal disease can have a recurrence if oral hygiene is not meticulous. By measuring the distance from the CEJ to the bottom of the pocket and from the top of the gingival margin to the bottom of the pocket, the hygienist can determine if the patient has gingival recession greater than expected for his/her age or if the patient has periodontal disease.

The examination

The hygienist examines the gingiva for color and texture. He/she also looks at gingival margins; are they smooth and knife-edged? Are they rounded, bulbous, or swollen? Is there bleeding when the probe is placed in the pocket? The hygienist, using a periodontal probe, measures the distance from the top of the gingival margin to the point the gingiva is attached to the tooth. The pocket (sulcus) depth indicates the extent of any gingival attachment. The hygienist, then, checks for mobility of the teeth by using two blunt-edged instruments to rock the tooth from facial to lingual. One blunt-edged instrument pressed on the incisal or occlusal surface indicates vertical mobility. The hygienist also looks for furcation involvement and occlusal trauma.

Mobility, recession, and furcation involvement

Mobility is documented by N for normal, 1 or I for slight horizontal mobility, 2 or II for moderate horizontal mobility greater than 1 mm, and 3 or III if the tooth moves in all directions. Furcation involvement is classified I for evidence of early bone loss in furcation area, II if the probe can enter the furca, III when the probe can pass completely through the furcation, and IV if the furcation is visible because of gingival recession. Recession is classified as from three points of view. Visible recession is measured from the CEJ to the gingival margin. Total or actual recession is the measurement from the CEJ to the base of the pocket, and apparent recession is a measurement of the visible root surface.

Charting

- *Carious lesions:* Usually primary teeth are lettered A – T with A being the upper right second primary molar and T being the lower right second primary molar. Permanent teeth are numbered 1 – 32 with 1 being the upper right third molar and 32 being the lower right third molar. A straight line or an X through the tooth on the chart indicates missing teeth. Black's Carious Lesion Classification denotes Class I as pits and fissures decay on occlusal, buccal, or lingual surfaces of posterior teeth or lingual surfaces of anterior teeth. Class II indicates decay on the proximal surface of molars and premolars. Class III denotes decay on the proximal surface of anterior teeth and cuspids. Class IV indicates decay on the proximal surface into the incisal edge of anterior teeth. Class V -- decay is on the cervical third of facial or lingual surfaces and Class VI indicates decay on a cusp tip.
- *Restorations:* All restorations are outlined, shaded, and labeled according to restorative material. Acrylic, composite resin, glass ionomer cements or porcelain, are charted with a blue outline and the letters C, CR, GIC, or R. Acrylic crowns are labeled AJC, and porcelain crowns, inlays, or veneers, are noted PJC, PI, or Ven. Porcelain fused to metal crowns are labeled PFM. Temporary restorations are labeled T. Sealants are charted with a blue S on the occlusal surface and amalgams are labeled A. Metal crowns are labeled FGC or GC for gold crown, ¾ GC for ¾ crowns. Onlays and inlays are labeled GO or GI. A pontic replaces a missing tooth in a bridge. The crown is labeled as other crowns but an X is placed on the root and double horizontal lines connect the pontic to the abutment crowns. Gold foil is labeled GF, and implants are charted as bridges with the label I.
- *Other items of interest:* New decay should be noted with a red outline and shading. Recurrent decay is charted with a red circle around existing restoration. Overhangs should be indicated in red. Supernumerary teeth should be drawn and noted Su. Congenitally missing teeth should be

labeled. Abrasion, abfraction, and attrition should be noted. Malposed teeth and open contacts should be indicated. Unerupted teeth usually are indicated with a circle around the unerupted part of the tooth. Root canals should be indicated (blue for present condition, red for diagnosed) with a line through the nerve chamber. Any other condition or item that is not usual for a patient of that age should be noted.

Causes of extrinsic stain

Stains and discolorations are usually documented with a written description. Many stains can be removed by scaling and polishing. Yellow stains usually indicate heavy plaque buildup. Black or black-line stains indicate iron compounds in oral fluids in patients with good oral hygiene. Orange stains are usually the result of chromogenic bacteria. Green stains at the cervical area can become intrinsic if oral hygiene is not improved and plaque removed daily. This stain is frequently accompanied by decalcified enamel. Tobacco, coffee, cola, and tea stains are brown to black and can be removed if they are not left there too long. Some antibacterial mouth rinses and some antibiotics leave brown or gray stains on teeth. Gray-green stain is usually associated with marijuana use.

Causes of endogenous stains

Endogenous stains are those that are a part of the tooth and can only be reduced by internal bleaching. Gray or brown intrinsic stains are frequently caused by tetracycline consumption during the time the teeth were developing. Fluoride in drinking water in greater concentrations than the recommended 0.7 ppm to 1.2 ppm can cause brown or white spots and sometimes pitting. Traumatized tooth pulp turns purple or black as it dies due to blood leaching into the dentin. Genetic tooth variance such as amelogenesis imperfecta causes white opaque teeth, and dentinogenesis can cause the teeth to look translucent blue. Hypocalcification cause the teeth to look opaque white, and porphyria cause teeth to look dark yellow or brown. Dentin dysplasia causes primary teeth to look blue.

Deposits on teeth

Bacterial plaque that is not removed hardens into hard, rock-like deposits called calculus. It is composed of minerals (mainly calcium phosphate, with some calcium carbonate and other organic compounds) that originate in saliva and fluid from the sulcus. Deposits are classified by their location, Supragingival calculus is attached to the crown of the tooth down to the gingival margin. When dry, it is chalky white; when wet, it is colored much like the tooth. Subgingival calculus is found below the gingival margin down to the bottom of the sulcus. It is usually dark brown to black. Subgingival calculus contributes to periodontal disease because it is porous and harbors bacteria. It irritates the gingiva and makes removing plaque uncomfortable as well as difficult.

Oral Evaluation

Palpation

The intra-oral examination consists of observation and palpation of structures of the oral cavity according to Brian and Cooper. The intra-oral examination begins with visual observation of color, texture, and change of size, color, or texture of intra-oral tissues followed by palpation of tissues for density and stability of underlying tissues. Each part of the oral tissue is compared with the corresponding tissue on the opposite side by squeezing tissue between thumb and finger or two fingers. The patient should extend the tongue and say "aah" so that the HCW can see the tonsils and the back of the throat. The floor of the mouth and tongue should be palpated for underlying cysts or tumors. The tongue should be held with one gauze square and drawn out and to the side to see and evaluate the ventral surface of the tongue. Any discrepancy between right and left sides and anything unusual should be documented and pointed out to the examining dentist for further evaluation.

Visual inspection

Visual inspections are part of an intra-oral exam. Lips should be checked for changes in size, cracking, and limited motion associated with stroke, Bell's palsy, etc. Labial and alveolar mucosa should be examined for ulcerated lesions, frenum attachment, and lesions associated with tobacco use. Buccal mucosa should be checked for abnormal lesions. Gingiva should be examined for texture, color, swelling and exudate, recession, and trauma from aggressive tooth brushing. The hard and soft palate may present tori, petechiae associated with systemic disease, or rash caused by nicotine or denture problems and function of the tongue. Each tissue examined should be checked for trauma from accident or abuse. Each finding should be documented and changes noted if the condition was present at the last examination.

Lesions on tongue

Small wart-like lesions are not uncommon, but they should be examined and excised. These papillomas, with a cauliflower-like surface, probably have well-defined borders. They are found on tongue, lips, buccal mucosa, gingiva, and the palate. They are raised, sometimes pedunculated, continuous layers of stratified squamous epithelium with thin, central connective tissue cores.

There are other benign lesions of the oral cavity than can cause the patient concern. Pigmented nevi (moles) in the oral cavity can be similar to those on other parts of the body. The intradermal nevi can appear smooth and flat or elevated. Junctional nevi, compound nevi, juvenile melanoma (Spitz nevus), and blue nevus should be watched from appointment to appointment for changes. Leukoplakia and leukoedema are white plaque on the mucosa. Leukoplakia is the more serious because it originates from chronic irritation or vitamin deficiency and can become malignant.

Tori

Tori are significant and can present problems for the patient who wears a partial or full denture. They should be removed if they interfere with denture wearing. Since a full maxillary denture depends on a tight seal to remain in place, tori can interfere when they grow to the back of the hard palate and do not allow the denture to seal properly. Lower dentures are notorious for being hard to keep in place because the seal is broken each time the patient swallows, talks, or moves the muscles under the tongue. If the patient has exostosis, the denture must be made short enough or wide enough to prevent irritation and a good seal is almost impossible to obtain.

Occlusal Evaluation

Importance of an occlusal evaluation

The relationship of the maxillary teeth to the mandibular teeth affects the esthetic appearance of the face, but more importantly, that relationship can affect the general health of the patient. Malposed teeth can make eating difficult or painful. Clenching and grinding in an attempt to make the teeth fit together damages the teeth and, sometimes, the temporomandibular joint. Headaches are a common complaint for the patient who has a poor relationship between maxillary and mandibular teeth. Dr. Edward Angle devised a classification system that provides guidance for correcting occlusal relationships when they inhibit eating, or other lifestyle choices. Guidelines are also provided for intervention when the dentist examines a child with primary malocclusion or malocclusion of mixed dentition.

Angle's Classification of Malocclusion

Dr. Edward Angle devised the most widely used classification system for occlusion based on the relationship of the first molars. Normal relationship places the mesiobuccal cusp of the maxillary first molar in the buccal groove of the mandibular first molar. The maxillary cuspid is in the facial embrasure of the mandibular first premolar and cuspid. Class II presents the mesiobuccal cusp of the first maxillary molar one cusp width mesial of the buccal groove of the mandibular first molar. Division I presents mandibular incisors retruded and maxillary incisors protruded. Division II presents the laterals more forward than centrals and maxillary incisors retruded. With Class III occlusion the mesiobuccal cusp of the first maxillary molar is one cusp width distal of the buccal groove of the mandibular first molar.

Clinical Testing

Tests provide information for better treatment planning and dental care. Plaque indexes can provide an effective visual indication of the amount of plaque that the patient is missing when he/she brushes and flosses. A colored fluid is used by the patient to rinse, and then he/she can see the plaque on the teeth. Lab tests to determine which specific bacterium is causing the periodontal disease gives the patient and the hygienist clues to which mouth rinse to use or which medication to place in the pocket for best results. Pulp vitality testing sometimes exposes pulp necrosis that is invisible to average oral examinations. Pulp vitality testing equipment can be battery-operated or can be plugged into an electrical outlet. The plug-ins are more dependable, but they must be used near an electrical outlet. This equipment should not be used with patients who wear pacemakers or other electronic life support.

Obtaining and Interpreting Radiographs

Radiographs

In addition to the visual and physical exam, the dentist needs radiographic images to see the areas between the teeth (the interproximal and contact areas). Frequently decay starts in areas that are inaccessible to toothbrushes and oral rinses. Patient compliance is sporadic, and the areas most often neglected are the contacts and subgingival areas. The radiographic image can expose those areas for close examination for incipient decay or decalcified areas. Normal tooth enamel is radiopaque. Dentin is more opaque than the root (nerve) chamber, and the root chamber is slightly more, or equally, opaque than bone structure of the jaw. As the tooth structure decalcifies, the tooth becomes more radiolucent, and allows the dentist to visualize the extent and significance of any decay. Radiographs also allow the dentist to monitor bone loss from periodontal disease, developmental anomalies, and occult disease.

The following components of an x-ray machine:

- The X-Ray tube, a glass-lined vacuum tube, has a cathode-negative electrode with a tungsten filament to provide electrons when heated. It has a semicircular molybdenum cup which is the anode-positive electrode to produce heat and x-rays. The copper stem with an embedded anode dissipates excessive heat. The focal spot is the target for the electrons.
- The power supply provides energy through a wire directly in one direction (DC) or alternating (AC) in first one direction, then the other. It is measured in amperes (milliamperes in dentistry) and uses voltage (kilovolts) as the unit of force between two points.
- The circuit is the route the electrical current moves through filament or in high-voltage. The filament circuit adjusts current through low-voltage circuits and controls the heating of the filament and availability of electrons by milliamperage (mA) setting. The high-voltage circuit uses 65,000 to 100,000 volts to provide voltage necessary to produce x-rays.

Measurement units for radiation

Traditional or standard units of measurement are Roentgen, rad, and rem. The international units are C/kg and gray sievert. The exposure dose is measured immediately before entering the patient's skin and tissues, and indicates the quantity of radiation and its ability to ionize the air. The Roentgen is the amount of radiation capable of ionizing 1.6 x 10^{n} (ten to the twelfth power) ion pairs per gram of air. The absorbed dose measures the quantity of any type of ionizing radiation (1 rad=.01 gray; 1 gray = 100 rads). Dose equivalent is the damage an individual might expect from different types of radiation. Rem (Roentgen equivalent man) = .01 sievert. All units may be written in smaller units (mRem = millirem).

Determining length of time necessary to produce quality X-Ray images

Amperage is the volume of electricity carried in a conductor. It is affected by the pressure of the current (the voltage) and the ohms (the resistance). Dental X-Ray machines measure volume of electricity in milliamps; current is measured in kilovolts; and resistance is measured in ohms. Greater numbers of X-Rays, or greater milliamperes, sent through the tube results in shorter exposure times. Longer, more penetrating, X-Rays require shorter exposure time. Intensifier screens reduce the exposure time, a shorter distance of the subject to the tube means shorter exposure, and a thicker and denser subject requires longer exposure. The sensitivity of the film affects necessary exposure as well. Now most extra-oral X-Ray machines are set at 60 or 70 kVp and 10 mA with variable exposure time for the usual Series E film. Exposure time or kVp may be increased for a large patient with denser bone structure.

How digital radiography systems operate

Digital operating systems vary regarding development time, but generally digital radiographs take about 90 seconds to 3 minutes to go to the computer compared to 3 to 5 minutes of developing time for traditional films. Semi-direct imaging stores the image on phosphor storage plates (PSP) which are then placed in a closed container (scanner) and exposed to laser light. The laser stimulates the PSP and records the light photons reflected. After the image has been sent to the computer, the PSP is exposed to high intensity light (light box) to completely clean the plate. The direct sensor system is connected to the computer by fiber optic wires which make the sensor (charge coupled device) bulky. However this system saves time and allows the operator to view the images immediately and retake images if necessary.

Advantages of using digital radiography

Contrary to early beliefs that digital radiology systems expose the patient to less radiation, the digital system exposure is about the same as with traditional systems. However the advantage of image manipulation definitely makes these systems worthwhile. Contrast enhancement allows the dentist to compensate for too light or too dark images. Calipers, rulers, and protractors provide opportunities for orthodontists and endodontists to measure exactly the parts of the tooth being treated. The dentist can also superimpose images onto other digital photographs to present end of case changes. Filtration and 3-D imaging allows results of reconstruction and proposed changes to be viewed. Of course, savings of time and storage space are obvious, and teleradiology facilitates sharing images between specialists and primary care dentists.

Disadvantages of using digital radiography

The most obvious disadvantage for using digital systems is the cost. Traditional systems must be modified for digital imaging or replaced completely. This cost should be compared with value of time saved and storage space not used for radiographs. The bulkiness of the sensor and the inconvenience of adjusting trailing wires should be considered as well. However, most patients will accept the inconvenience when they realize the advantages of seeing images immediately and manipulating images for ease of diagnosis. Cross-contamination can be awkward because the sensor must be placed in a plastic bag and wiped down for each patient. If the sensor does become directly contaminated, the sensor should be discarded and replaced regardless of cost. There is also the possibility of digital images being manipulated for fraudulent purposes. Software manufacturers are now providing tracking provisions that retrieve the original image if necessary.

Principles of Radiologic Health

Sources of radiation exposure

Natural background radiation from the earth's atmosphere, gamma rays from rocks and soil, radon, and its decay products, and ingested radioisotopes from certain foods comprise about 82% of the radiation to which patients are exposed. Artificial background radiation in the form of fallout from nuclear explosions and radioactive waste make up less than .1% of exposure to radiation. Occupational exposure comprises less than 1%, and medical and dental diagnostic radiation accounts for the remaining 18% of usual exposure. Many patients are wary of having dental radiographs exposed because of fear of too much radiation; however, dental and medical radiation from a properly adjusted and maintained X-Ray unit delivers a very small amount of radiation compared to the benefits that the diagnostic films provide for good dental treatment,

Radiation biology and how it interacts with matter

Radiation biology is the study of the effects of radiation on living matter. Attenuation is the way radiation is absorbed as it passes through the subject. The X-Rays lose their energy as they pass through matter and scatter (Compton scattering). As it reaches the subject, the X-Ray photon gives an outer electron to the outer shell of the subject causing ionization. Colliding photons scatter is various directions. About 62% of the photons that leave the tube scatter, and about 30% of the scatter escapes the subject tissue. About 30% of the photons leaving the X-Ray beam are absorbed by the patient and do not fog the film. About 9% of the X-Rays cause an interaction, and less than 8% of the energy scatters close enough to excite absorber atoms, but not close enough to affect the patient or the film.

Effects of radiation on living cells

Radiation energy is absorbed by molecules and transferred between unstable molecules. Unstable molecules are rearranged so that they have different structure and function from original form, but they become stable and set a new pattern. The direct effect accounts for about 1/3 of the damaged molecules created by radiation. The other biological damage (about 2/3) is an indirect effect producing free radicals, such as hydroxyl, that form new molecules with different chemical and biological properties. Linear transfer energy causes more damage than radiation. Somatic cell sensitivity includes cancer and other disorders that do not involve genetic tissues. Genetic effects are passed on to future generations with possible mutated cells. No dose of radiation is safe. The Law of Bergonie-Tribondeau describes mitotic activity, growth cells, undifferentiated cells, and cells with a large nucleus as being most sensitive to the effects of radiation.

Guidelines for safely exposing diagnostic radiographs

The first rule of thumb is to use X-Ray settings as low as reasonably possible (ALARA). Each radiograph should produce a benefit greater than the risk. There should be a need determined by the patient history and clinical findings, and the up-to-date equipment should be the best that is available to produce diagnostic images with the lowest possible exposure. Film speed E reduces exposure time by about 40% to 50% compared to D, and F reduces exposures by 20% more. Correct positioning with film holders and quality processing reduce necessary retakes. The patient should be protected by using lead shields that have a layer of lead at least .25mm thick. The thyroid collar and aprons protect the patient from secondary, reflected radiation.

Cell and tissue sensitivity

Tissue sensitivity is categorized from radiosensitive to radio-resistant. Cells with the highest sensitivity are small lymphocytes, bone marrow, reproductive cells, and intestinal mucosa. These cells replicate very quickly, and some have little or no specialized function. Connective tissue, small blood vessels, growing bone and cartilage, salivary glands, lungs, kidneys, and liver cells are categorized as being intermediately sensitive. They can be easily damaged, but being differentiated, they can still function. Optic lens, mature erythrocytes, muscle, and nerve cells are the most differentiated and the least sensitive to radiation damage. There are several somatic tissues that, when damaged, function improperly. Though they do not pass the damage to future generations, critical organs such as female breast, skin, thyroid, and hematopoietic tissues can cease to function properly after too much radiation. The radiation injury can accumulate beyond repair of the organ.

Technique

Exposure technique and the processing quality

The darkroom should be designed with good ventilation and no light leaks. Since white light destroys the image on the film before fixing, every effort should ensure that no white light enters the darkroom during processing. A red or orange light does not affect film quality. The temperature should be about 70°F/21°C; humidity should be between 50% and 70%; and the area should be immaculately clean. The processing chemicals should be refreshed daily and old chemicals should be replaced every two weeks to four weeks, or more often if film quality becomes too light. The developer reduces silver halide crystals to make the image apparent. The rinsing solution (water) stops development and removes excess chemicals from the emulsion. The fixer removes unexposed halide crystals. Washing again removes excess chemicals, and drying removes excess water.

Manual versus automatic processing

Manual processing is time consuming (about 30 – 35 minutes) compared with automatic processors (4.5 to 5.5 minutes). The operator must watch each step closely and time each part of the process in order to avoid overdeveloping or under washing or under fixing the film. The film can be viewed after about three minutes, but the image is not completely fixed for about seven more minutes. Temperature of the developer and development time are directly related – warmer developer temperature shortens development time, but it can reduce diagnostic quality, making films dark. There is also a greater possibility that chemicals can be spilled or exposed to air.

Automatic processing provides a closed system for the chemicals, providing less deterioration from exposure to air. The operator can use daylight loaders or a darkroom for placing films in the processor and can leave to continue patient treatment if necessary.

Parallel technique

The parallel technique of dental radiography works on the principle of placing the film parallel to the long axis of the tooth. There are various film holders available for purchase, but the most widely used are the Rinn rings. This system provides a plastic tab that fits on a metal arm. The patient bites on the tab which holds the film parallel to the long axis of the tooth. The metal arm holds a ring, outside the patient's mouth, which provides a focus for the X-Ray cone. The hygienist places the flat plane of the opening of the cone parallel to the ring which is parallel to the long axis of the tooth and the flat plane of the film in the patient's mouth. The X-Ray beam is activated; the film is removed and processed.

Traditional and digital radiography

In traditional radiography the silver halide emulsion on the film acts as radiation detector and image display. In digital radiography, the image is composed of light sensitive elements (pixels) which display on the computer screen. Direct imaging places the image directly from the X-Ray machine to the computer using an intra-oral sensor similar to the traditional film and film holder. After it is on the computer screen, the image can be manipulated to improve contrast or density, or it can be retaken. Semi-direct imaging places the image on a phosphor storage plate (similar to conventional film) which is then placed in a receptacle where it is scanned by a laser that stores the image on the computer.

Assuring quality radiographs

The best quality radiographs should have clear images with no fogging of subject and no artifacts. The X-Ray machine should be tested at recommended intervals by qualified service personnel for radiation output, timer accuracy, milliamperage reproducibility, and collimation. The kilovoltage should be calibrated at that time. The arm should be tested for drifting and tightened when necessary. Darkroom conditions should be monitored closely. Safelight filters and distance should be examined, and any light leaks should be eliminated with black masking tape or weather stripping. Daily testing of processing efficiency is advised as well. Film should be stored in a cool, dry area away from the X-Ray source. Cassettes should be examined monthly for defects, lead aprons should be checked for breaks in the lead lining, and the viewbox should be inspected. Viewbox lights should be replaced when needed, and the viewbox should be cleaned routinely as part of the operatory sanitation.

Normal and Abnormal Radiographs

Recognizing an abnormal situation on dental radiographic film

First, the hygienist must have a thorough knowledge of the normal anatomical landmarks. The hygienist should know the relative density of the structures and how they should look on a radiograph. Time and experience help the hygienist to learn how some of the most common artifacts look and how they are produced in order to avoid producing the artifacts in practice. The hygienist should learn what incipient decay looks like, what supernumerary teeth look like, and how the mandibular canal and mental foramen appear on radiographs. Careful study provides invaluable information, and practice at identifying anatomical landmarks and abnormalities are the best ways for the hygienist to learn to "read" radiographs.

Example: A young adult patient arrives at the dental office for his twice-yearly dental prophylaxis. He reports no problems and wants to hurry through this routine exam so the hygienist proceeds immediately to expose four bitewing radiographs and a panoramic film. The hygienist notices a radiopaque lump on the dorsal surface of the patient's tongue.

First, the hygienist should ask the patient if he is wearing tongue jewelry as she should have asked before taking the pano. Even when the patient wants to hurry through the appointment, removing jewelry before panoramic radiographs saves time. If the patient is wearing tongue jewelry, he must remove it so that the hygienist can take a diagnostic radiograph. If the patient is not wearing tongue jewelry, the hygienist should proceed with the extra-oral and intra-oral exam to collect as much information as possible for the exam and diagnosis by the dentist. Careful examination of the tongue and surrounding areas is important for a good diagnosis. If the "lump" is not jewelry, every effort should be made to identify the object and decide if a referral to a specialist is advisable.

<u>Interpretation versus diagnosis</u>

Debralee Nelson defined interpretation as "the means of explaining or clarifying what is seen on a dental radiograph." She defines diagnosis as "the specific identification of a condition or disease by examination, or a conclusion drawn from symptoms." She also reminds the hygienist that only dentists diagnose a problem. The hygienist can examine the oral structures and, with the recommendation of the dentist, expose radiographs for further examination of the teeth and periodontal tissues. The hygienist can look for radiolucencies between the teeth, at occlusal surfaces or buccal or lingual pits, and on root surfaces that indicate possible carious lesions. He/she can then call the attention of the dentist to these abnormalities.

<u>Periodontal disease</u>

Periodontal disease is an assortment of abnormalities affecting the structures that support the teeth. Gingivitis is an inflammation of the gingiva presenting swelling, bleeding, and tenderness. It is frequently caused by poor oral hygiene;

sometimes medications and/or hormonal imbalance cause sensitivity and bleeding. Gingivitis can usually be controlled by excellent oral hygiene. Continued symptoms of gingivitis, after oral hygiene has improved, indicate the possibility of a systemic disorder causing the dentist to refer the patient to his/her primary care physician.

Periodontitis is inflammation that involves the alveolar bone and leads to bone loss and mobile, or lost, teeth. The first radiographic indication of periodontitis is a fuzzy area around the cortical crest of bone. As the disease progresses, vertical or horizontal bone loss appears. The progress of periodontitis is measured by considering bone loss, overhanging margins of restorations, the presence of caries, calculus, and root resorption and periapical lesions.

Trauma changes, resorption, and pulpal and periapical lesions

Trauma results from falls or blows to the face or mouth. Occasionally the trauma is sufficient to completely remove the tooth from the bone. Resorption occurs when the tooth structure is lost with no visible clinical recognition. External resorption begins at the root and exhibits a flat apical tip radiographically. Internal resorption begins in the pulp and moves into the dentin as a result of trauma or pulp capping. Pulp stones are round, radiopaque calcification in the pulp of molars. Pulp erasure is the disappearance of the pulp chamber due to trauma. The pulp disappears as secondary dentin forms in the pulp canals. Periapical lesions can be caused by an abscess around the tip of the root or a radiolucent granuloma on the tip. Condensing osteitis is associated with a low-grade infection and sclerotic bone is most often associated with inflammation.

Planning/Managing Dental Hygiene

Infection Control

Infection control protocol

Each patient has a different set of medical conditions that may, or may not, interfere with optimal health. The condition that may not interfere with one patient's health may be life-threatening for another. The bacteria that are balanced for one patient may be totally unbalanced for another. A dental health worker can spread (cross-contaminate) bacteria from one patient to another if care is not taken to completely sanitize the operatory and sterilize instruments after each patient's treatment. Following a carefully written plan for sanitizing the operatory and sterilizing equipment provides the health care worker with the best chance of preventing cross-contamination between patients and between the health care worker and the patient. Using approved personal protective equipment protects the health care worker from aerosols and other routes of contamination.

PPE recommended by CDC

Personal protective equipment (PPE) is designed to protect the skin and the mucous membranes of the eyes, nose, and mouth of dental health-care personnel from exposure to blood or other potentially infectious material".
PPE should be moisture proof and used for only one patient. Masks prevent aerosols from entering the respiratory system. Safety glasses that cover the eyebrows to the cheekbones and have side shields protect the worker from aerosols as well as splashes of oral fluids. Lab jackets that fasten at the throat and reach past the hips protect clothing. The jackets should have sleeves that protect the arms from circulating aerosol bacteria and have cuffs that can be tucked into the cuffs of latex, vinyl, or nitrile disposable gloves. Each of these

items protects the dental health care worker in the office and prevents the worker from inadvertently taking bacteria home to family.

Sanitizing

The hygienist enters the operatory and removes all jewelry. After a three-minute hand scrub, the hygienist puts on personal protective equipment and scrubs down the chair and counters with an approved sanitizing solution. He/she runs the air/water syringe and the slow-speed hand piece for one minute and cycles disinfecting solution through electronic scalers to clear any bacteria from the lines. He/she replaces the disinfecting solution with distilled water in the closed system. Barriers are placed on light handles, drawer pulls, chairs, and any surface that can not be sanitized or sterilized. After replacing disposable gloves, the hygienist sets out the instruments and items needed for the specific patient. The hygienist then discards disposable PPE. After seating the patient, the hygienist, again, dons PPE before treating the patient.

After releasing the patient, the hygienist dons PPE including heavy utility gloves. Sharps are placed in specified containers, and biohazard items are properly discarded. Other disposable items and barriers are placed in a bag for disposal. Soiled instruments are placed on the tray for transfer to sterilization. The chair is wiped down with a solution appropriate for the care of the upholstery and sanitizing protocol. Hard surfaces are wiped down then sprayed with the sanitizing solution and left to air dry. The tray with all exposed instruments is covered and taken to sterilizing area. Instruments are rinsed and placed in the ultrasonic bath, with the lid closed, for five minutes to loosen debris and blood. After five minutes, the instruments are taken out of the ultrasonic bath, rinsed in running water, and air-dried before packaging with a steri-strip. Packages are placed loosely in the autoclave and sterilized according to manufacturer's instructions.

Sterilizing instruments

Moist heat uses steam under pressure to kill spores, tubercule bacillus, and other contaminants. This is useful for all instruments that can withstand the 250˚F temperatures for the required 20 minutes at about 15 psi. The disadvantages include corrosion and/or melting of instruments not designed for steam autoclaving and the inability of steam to penetrate oils and powders.

Dry heat sterilizes by oxidation and is effective for oils and powders and for instruments that corrode. It preserves sharp edges of instruments, but it requires 1 to 2 hours at 320˚F at 30 psi.

Chemical vapor uses combinations (alcohol, formaldehyde, ketone, acetone, and water) to penetrate packaging. It requires the manufacturer's chemical solution, but it provides rust and corrosion-free operation, 20 minutes at 270˚F at 20 – 40 psi, and quick drying. A disadvantage is the toxic chemical vapor. Quick turn-around sterilizers are effective at 375˚F for 8 – 12 minutes.

Standards for office safety

"Dental offices must have a written, comprehensive safety plan to protect patients and staff from infectious disease" These precautions apply to employees at risk for occupational exposure, but every employee should be familiar with the plan. Briefly, these are information and training for employees, use of universal precautions by every at risk employee, determination of which employees are at risk, HBV vaccination for employees at risk for exposure, provision of appropriate personal protective equipment for everyone in the treatment area, periodic office cleaning and decontamination, evaluation and follow up of occupational exposures, maintenance of accurate medical records after occupational exposures, and labeling of all containers of regulated waste with a biohazard label.

Preparing for emergency situations

The best way to prepare for any emergency situation is training and practice and knowing patient histories well enough to watch for subtle warning signs. CPR training and certification are required for all dental hygienists before they can be licensed. This training must be updated every two years by the American Heart Association or the American Red Cross. Dental offices should have a written procedure detailing the duties of each member of the emergency response team for that office. Emergency situations should be practiced regularly so that when a situation arises, each member of the team feels comfortable that he/she knows exactly what to do and does it automatically.

If the office staff does not participate in daily review of charts for each scheduled patient, the hygienist should review the charts for his/her patients and consult the dentist for any questionable entries. Being alert for possible problems improves patient care.

Preventing common emergencies

Syncope, or fainting, is the most common emergency in the dental office. Like other emergency situations in which the patient is unconscious, syncope can lead to airway obstruction and death if not properly treated. Fainting causes blood flow to the brain to decrease. Stress is the usual cause, but poor health, exhaustion, and postural hypotension are possible causes. Recognizing the signs that indicate a pre-syncope stage and stopping treatment can prevent most syncope episodes. The patient, who is about to faint, feels dizzy and/or nauseous and looks pale, breathing becomes shallow and pupils dilate before the patient loses consciousness. The patient should be placed in the Trendelenburg position, or if pregnant, on her side. The hygienist should insure an open airway and carefully use an ammonia inhalant to stimulate breathing. The patient might need oxygen, but the patient always needs to be monitored until vital signs return to normal.

First aid kit or crash cart

There are five essential items for the crash cart. The resuscitation mask or face shield with a one-way valve provides a means to supply oxygen to the patient who has fainted or is breathing on his/her own. Oxygen with a positive pressure ventilation capability or an Ambu bag forces oxygen into the lungs of a patient who is not breathing on his/her own. Nitroglycerin tablets (0.3 mg) or an oral nitroglycerin spray relieves angina pain. Tablets have a shelf life of about six months and oral spray has a longer shelf life. Frequent evaluation of all items in the kit (or on the cart) will insure the effectiveness of all medicines. Epinephrine (two preloaded 1:1,000 syringes) stimulates the heart, constricts blood vessels, dilates bronchioles, and elevates blood glucose. An injectable antihistamine such as Benadryl or Chlor-Trimeton treats an allergic reaction.

Most dental offices want the first aid kit or crash cart to have some supplies in addition to those necessary for basic emergencies. Amyl nitrate vaporole is a vasodilator used as an inhalant to treat angina. Anti-asthmatic bronchodilators are used specifically to open bronchioles and relieve discomfort of asthma attacks. Aromatic ammonia vaporoles are frequently taped to the light fixture for use immediately if the patient faints. Gauze, bandages, and adhesive tape are used more by staff for minor accidents than for patients. Oral sucrose is administered to patients who experience low blood sugar while in the dental chair. Syringes and tourniquets are useful for staff accidents as well as patient treatment.

Basic life support

The steps to deliver basic life support to a patient in the dental office: Determine unconsciousness – Shake the patient gently. Activate EMS. Position the patient on a hard surface. Open the airway with head-tilt, chin-lift method. (A) Determine if the patient is breathing for 7 to 15 seconds. (B) Ventilate twice with each breath lasting about two seconds. Check for a pulse (C-cardiac) at the carotid artery for 5 – 10 seconds. Locate the landmark at the lower end of the sternum with two fingers. Place the heel of the other hand on the landmark. Place the first hand on top of the second hand with the fingers elevated. Press down about 1½ to 2 inches being careful to keep the hand in contact with the patient's chest. Give 15 compressions and give 2 breaths. Repeat the process for one minute and reassess pulse and breathing until the patient's heart begins to beat and the patient breathes voluntarily or another trained person takes over.

CPR with two rescuers

The second rescuer should identify himself as being trained in CPR. He calls EMS if the first rescuer has not done so. He checks the patient's pulse for 5 – 10 seconds and replies that pulse is or is not present. He then changes places with the first rescuer. The first rescuer observes results of rescue breaths and checks for a pulse between compressions. Cycles of 2 breaths and 15 compressions continue, providing 80 to 100 compressions and about 12 breaths each minute. "...If the heart is in fibrillation, defibrillation is necessary to make compressions effective" (Nelson, 2000). Defibrillators are now a common part of most commercially prepared first aid kits, and training for using defibrillators is a part of CPR training.

CPR for adult, child and infant

CPR for a child patient (one to eight years) differs from the adult in a couple of ways. Fibrillation of a child patient's heart is uncommon; since most of the time, the child patient goes into cardiac arrest because of respiratory difficulty. If there is only one rescuer present, the rescuer performs CPR for one minute, and then EMS is called. CPR technique for the child is the same as for an adult except that the heel of only one hand is used for compressions rather than two. Compressions are 1 to 1½ inches and five compressions are followed by one breath per three seconds or about 20 cycles per minute.

CPR for an infant less than one year old is also different from that for an adult. The infant is turned on his back with his head and neck supported during the turn. The look, listen, and feel routine is performed before rescue breathing is begun. The rescuer's mouth should cover the infant's nose and mouth, and breaths should last about 1 to 1½ seconds each. Pulse is checked for about five seconds at the brachial artery on the inside of the infant's arm. Compressions are given with the middle finger and the ring finger on the infant's sternum at a depth of ½ to 1 inch. Five compressions are given for each breath at the rate of at least 100 compressions per minute. After one minute pulse and breathing are assessed, and CPR is continued until help arrives or the infant's pulse returns.

Grand mal seizures

Seizures can be caused by a systemic disorder such as epilepsy or from prolonged high fever, alcohol or drug withdrawal, trauma, congenital abnormalities, or an imbalance of body fluids. Grand mal seizures are the most common type, especially for patients with epilepsy. The prodromal phase, the first phase, may include a personality change, an aura that is unique for that person, and may last a few seconds to several hours. The convulsive or ictal phase includes a loss of consciousness, an epileptic cry as air rushes from the lungs, and tonic (rigid body) and clonic (relaxed body) movements. This phase lasts about 2 – 5 minutes. The postictal phase occurs after tonic-clonic movements and last 10 – 30 minutes in which the patient sleeps. Monitoring the patient and providing basic life support when necessary is vital for patient survival. The patient usually wakes confused and disoriented before full recovery.

Seizures

Petit mal seizures (absence seizures) present a loss of awareness for a few seconds and occur more frequently in children than in adults. The patient stares blankly and may experience minor twitching or rapid blinking. Partial seizures are characterized by jerking on only one side because only a part of the brain is affected. These seizures present a trance-like appearance and purposeless activity. Hysterical seizures occur when there is an audience, are usually manipulation techniques triggered by emotional upset. These movements are usually more controlled. Status epilepticus presents the same characteristics as other seizures, but it lasts longer than five minutes, is uninterrupted, with no recovery between episodes. Status epilepticus is the major cause of death associated seizures. Main objective of treatment in the dental office is to prevent the patient from hurting himself.

Hyperglycemia

Hyperglycemic patients can have either type I (insulin dependent diabetes mellitus) or type II (non-insulin dependent diabetes mellitus). Type I diabetes is controlled with daily injections of insulin, and type II diabetes is usually controlled by diet and exercise, but type II may require medication such as Orinase or Glucophage. Insulin shock, or low blood sugar, occurs when a diabetic patient skips a meal, exercises more than usual, has excess insulin, or sometimes just changes his/her routine. Symptoms of low blood sugar include cold sweat, headache, trembling, weakness, a possible personality change, nervousness, and confusion. Administering a sugar source is the most efficient way to increase a patient's blood sugar. If the patient loses consciousness, glucagon should be administered intramuscularly. Seizure activity is more likely to occur if the patient is unconscious for longer than five minutes.

In an emergency, untreated hyperglycemia can lead to unconsciousness. Possible causes of emergency situations with hyperglycemic patients are non-compliance with therapy, infection, illness, or stress. Symptoms of hyperglycemia are increased thirst and urination, loss of appetite, nausea, vomiting, heavy breathing, dry warm skin, and a fruity, sweet odor of the breath. Tachycardia, and lower than usual blood pressure are indicative of hyperglycemia. If the patient begins to experience these symptoms, dental treatment should stop and EMS should be called. If there is a question of whether the patient is hyperglycemic or hypoglycemic, the patient should have a sugar source while waiting for EMS. Serious damage or death occurs more quickly for untreated hypoglycemic patients than for untreated hyperglycemic patients.

Common dental emergencies

Dry socket, traumatic displaced or avulsed teeth, acute pericornitis, postsurgical bleeding, and broken instruments, are possible emergency situations in the dental office. Dry socket occurs when the patient displaces the blood clot that "bandages" an extraction site. A medicated dressing is placed daily until the site heals enough that the bone is no longer exposed. Displaced or avulsed teeth can be caused by trauma from many sources. The patient should keep the tooth in milk or in his cheek until the dentist can replace it and splint it. Acute pericornitis occurs when gingiva around an erupting tooth becomes infected. Irrigation with a warm salt water rinse soothes the gingiva, and an antibiotic prescription reduces lymphadenopathy and fever. Postsurgical bleeding is treated by pressure on the site with gauze packs or tea bags. Broken instruments should be removed as carefully as possible to prevent pieces from being swallowed by the patient.

Individualized Patient Education

Beginning education

The hygienist should first establish a rapport with the patient if possible. This rapport can begin with the greeting and continue to build throughout the appointment. The hygienist should consider the patient's physical age and his capacity to understand instructions. For example, the hygienist should not explain how to brush his teeth to a six-year-old using the same words that he/she would use when explaining to an adult. Generally, conversation for a few minutes with the patient will provide necessary clues to the patient's language comprehension level. A review with the patient of the patient's medical and dental history will usually give clues to the patient's attitude toward medical and dental care and his particular home care.

<u>Example:</u> The six-year-old patient dances into the operatory with a big smile on her face and hops into the dental chair. Looking at her chart and again at the child, the hygienist asks her mom if this is the same patient who would not open her mouth six months ago when she was present for a check-up. The mom confirms that this is the same patient, but now the child is eager to have her teeth cleaned and examined.

Six-year-old children vary in their willingness to cooperate with any particular procedure. Since the previous appointment was a pleasant experience, and she was not forced to allow the oral prophylaxis after the hygienist confirmed with the parent that there were no dental problems, the child had no negative feelings about seeing the hygienist again. The parents had encouraged good oral hygiene and promoted the next prophy appointment during the intervening six months as a "grown-up" experience. After assuring herself that no abuse contributed to the change in attitude, the hygienist should proceed with the appointment as if the new cooperation is simply a mark of growing maturity in the patient. A child who sings and dances her way into the dental operatory obviously likes music, so teaching her to floss and brush her teeth while music plays is a good way to build rapport. Showing the patient how to floss and to brush using a puppet with teeth and a large toothbrush lets her see the necessary action to clean all the teeth. Allowing her to practice brushing the puppet's teeth lets her feel the necessary action. Painting her teeth with disclosing solution and letting her brush the colored solution off the teeth translates the lesson into personal experience. The hygienist should suggest that the patient begin to brush her teeth at the beginning of a song and brush until that song ends so that she will have a definite idea of how long she should brush to get all the plaque and bacteria off her teeth each time she brushes.

Example: The truck-driver patient arrives for his regular six month prophy. During the examination, he says that he does not have time to floss his teeth every day.

Ask the patient if he has to wait at the dock while his truck is being loaded. If he says yes, then suggest that he use that waiting time to use floss picks that he keeps in the glove box of his truck. If he says that his truck is already loaded when he gets to the dock, then suggest that he use the time that he waits at stop lights to floss. If he watches television, the patient can keep floss picks near his chair to floss while he watches television. The objective to this lesson is to get the patient to start thinking about the short periods of time in his day when he is not busy. Floss picks are not as effective as string floss, but they do disturb plaque and bacteria if they are used daily.

Teaching patients to floss

The hygienist asks the patient to hold up his hand with the thumb toward the patient's chest. The hygienist tells the patient that his hand represents a row of teeth. The hygienist shows the patient how to wrap the floss, catching the end under the second wrap, on the middle finger of his/her non-dominant hand and the remainder of the 12 – 18 inch floss on the middle finger of the dominant hand. He/she explains that the dominant hand serves as the supply and the non-dominant hand serves as the take-up for the floss. Then the hygienist shows the patient how to slide the floss through the contact (fingers representing teeth) point, wrap the floss in a C-shape, and scrape the side of the tooth as the floss is removed. As time permits, the hygienist observes the patient practicing the lesson first on the hygienist's hands and then on his own teeth.

Extra-oral exam explanation

As he/she performs each element of the extra-oral exam, the hygienist tells the patient what he/she is doing. Palpating the lymph nodes reveals any sub-acute problems such as infection in the areas that those lymph nodes drain. Tenderness in the muscles near the ears indicates a possible ear infection or a malfunctioning temporomandibular joint. Tenderness of the facial muscles could indicate that the patient clenches or grinds his teeth during sleep. Observation that the patient's mouth does not open and close smoothly alerts the hygienist of probable TMJ dysfunction. Seeing a small open lesion on the patient's lip alerts the hygienist of immediate past or present fever and the need to postpone treatment until the herpes simplex outbreak is healed. Each element provides information that the hygienist and dentist need to treat that patient in the best way possible.

Intra-oral exam explanation

As he/she checks each part of the patient's mouth, the hygienist explains to the patient what he/she sees. For example, gingival recession could indicate that the patient brushes too hard, so the hygienist asks about brushing habits. Notches on the teeth immediately above the gingival margin could indicate grinding habits or brushing too hard. Bleeding gingiva alerts the hygienist to lack of flossing, use of some medications, hormone fluctuations, or a systemic disease that should be addressed by the dentist and/or the primary care physician. White, leathery patches indicate the probable use of tobacco products or possible pre-cancerous conditions. Each factor should be explained to the patient as it is found and documented in the permanent record. It is then called to the attention of the dentist during his/her exam.

Example: A patient arrives for a routine dental prophy and mentions that his lower left molar area has been sensitive to cold and sweets for the last two weeks.

Since the dentist has pre-authorized bite-wing radiographs twice each year, the hygienist should expose bite-wings as instructed. While the X-Rays are processing, the hygienist should continue with the preliminary exam and include pictures using the intra-oral camera. After they are taken, the hygienist should show the pictures to the patient and explain that the area will be brought to the dentist's attention. The hygienist should explain that sometimes, even with the best of care, bacteria gets into the occlusal grooves of molars and causes decay. The hygienist should explain that the dark areas in the grooves probably indicate that a carious lesion is present and that the dentist can remove the caries and restore the tooth. The hygienist should review flossing, brushing and rinsing instructions with the patient and reiterate the necessity of keeping a plaque-free oral environment through meticulous home care and regular dental check-ups.

Carious lesions

Bacteria which co-exist in a healthy mouth can get into grooves or pits of healthy teeth. If the pH of the oral environment drops below 5.5, the acidophilic bacteria proliferate and attack enamel. The acidic saliva begins to dissolve enamel, and bacteria destroy it, causing decay. Meticulous oral hygiene disturbs or removes the bacteria, and supplemental fluoride rinses help to re-mineralize the enamel. However, even though it is the hardest substance in the body, enamel can not resist dissolution if it is continuously bathed in an acidic solution with bacteria eating away. If it grows through the enamel, the lesion reaches the dentin. Dentin, about as dense as bone, transmits more sensitivity as the heat, cold, or sweets normally in the oral environment reach the nerve endings there.

Example: An adult patient arrives at the dental office for his regularly scheduled dental prophy. The intra-oral examination reveals that tooth #15 has a large, dark lesion on the mesiobuccal groove and a chipped mesiobuccal cusp. The interview reveals that the patient has had intermittent pain associated with cold and pressure for the last two weeks.

The hygienist should continue with the intra-oral examination, exposing radiographs as authorized by the dentist and asking questions about the instances and severity of the pain. The hygienist should review the etiology of carious lesions. Decay prevention by completely removing all plaque and disturbing and/or removing bacteria should also be reviewed. The hygienist might ask the patient about brushing habits and to demonstrate his brushing technique. The hygienist can correct insufficient cleaning habits only after he/she learns how the patient is cleaning his teeth and mouth. The hygienist should also ask the patient whether he crunches ice or eats popcorn kernels in order to assess the possibility of inadvertent cracking of teeth. The tooth could have had a hairline crack that allowed bacteria to invade and cause decay.

The hygienist should compliment his/her patient for the obvious good oral hygiene. The hygienist should explain that brushing does not reach the areas between the teeth to remove plaque and bacteria. Even though he flosses a couple of times each week, the patient is not getting the sides of his teeth and the contact areas clean. Only flossing, with the string scraping the sides of each tooth can disturb plaque and bacteria in the sulcus between the teeth. The hygienist should review flossing instructions, complete with a demonstration, with the patient. After the hygienist has demonstrated flossing, the patient should practice flossing his own teeth. The hygienist should emphasize that disturbing and removing plaque on a daily basis, in addition to brushing and rinsing, is the best way to prevent decay.

Periodontitis

The bacterial population of the human oral environment consists of thousands of bacteria balanced precariously between health and disease. Good oral hygiene, with daily plaque removal and a healthy immune system, keeps that balance unless the patient develops a systemic illness. If he develops a systemic illness, the patient's immune system sends white blood cells to the site of the injury or illness in an effort to fight off major disease. A lapse in good oral hygiene can allow bacteria to proliferate. As it builds on the tooth, the plaque migrates toward the apex of the root, dissolving periodontal fibers and irritating the gingiva. The plaque hardens into calculus, further irritating gingiva and causing bleeding. The immune system sends white blood cells to the site of the irritation causing swelling and further bleeding. The process can continue until bone has dissolved and teeth are loose or lost.

Example: A patient arrives for his perio maintenance appointment saying that he has noticed bleeding again when he brushes.

Bleeding gingiva is usually caused by bacterial imbalance in the oral environment, but occasionally, bleeding results from medication causing the imbalance or for incipient illness. During the extra-oral exam the hygienist should ask the patient about any systemic illnesses that he has or new problems that he has learned about since his last check-up. The hygienist should also ask about any new medications that the patient has begun to take since his last check-up. After verifying that the patient has no new medicines or illnesses, the hygienist should assess the efficacy of oral hygiene. The intra-oral exam will provide clues regarding oral hygiene. The hygienist should review oral hygiene instruction and suggest further tests to determine the need for treating with a perio chip or other antibiotic treatment.

Bleeding gingiva is usually the first sign of periodontal disease. Swollen gingiva results when the immune system sends white blood cells to the site of irritation or injury. The gingiva loses its sharp margins and begins to pull away from the teeth as plaque and/or calculus build up and migrate toward the root tip. These visible signs of disease can usually be reversed with close attention to cleaning the oral environment. As he/she continues with the intra-oral exam, the hygienist measures the distance from the top of the gingival margin to the point that the gingiva is attached to the tooth. This pocket depth indicates how well the patient can remove plaque from the teeth. The measurement from the cemento-enamel junction to the bottom of the pocket indicates the amount of gingival recession. Continued recession exposes root surfaces to the oral environment and increases the incidence of Class V caries.

Oral environment explanation

Bacteria thrive in a warm, moist environment. *Streptococcus mutans* initiate the decay process by breaking polysaccharides into lactic acid and *Lactobacillus acidophilus* extends the process. Any food particles left in the mouth can ferment and increase the acidic level of the saliva. An inadequate amount of saliva present influences the pH level and increases the incidence of decay by decreasing the pH. This decreased amount of saliva during sleep explains why dental health workers recommend cleaning the teeth thoroughly by brushing, flossing, and rinsing with an antibacterial rinse before bedtime. Between-meal snacking promotes decay by preventing the pH level from rising beyond 5.5 (the level at which demineralization begins). Dental health workers recommend brushing after between-meal snacks as well as after meals and before bedtime.

Calculus, materia alba, dental stains, faulty restorations, and impacted food are all factors that promote decay and periodontal disease. Plaque and calculus are the most obvious factors because they harbor bacteria that dissolve tooth enamel. However, materia alba is the first substance to adhere to teeth and attract bacteria. Unlike calculus, materia alba can be washed away with water, but it combines with bacteria and food debris and begins to harden within a short time. Food debris that is not brushed or washed away immediately sticks to the teeth and gingiva. Restorations that have begun to break down, and poorly fitted restoration margins, provide crevices and cracks in which bacteria thrive. Food or drink stains, though not as deep as cracks, provide a sticky surface to which bacteria cling. The sugars in saliva combine with any, or all, these other elements to destroy tooth enamel and cause gingival disease.

Anxiety, Pain Control, and Compromised Patients

Anxiety, fear, and phobia

Anxiety is uneasiness about the unknown; fear extrapolates anxiety, for known or unknown factors; phobia is uneasiness so excessive that it results in lack of action. The hygienist who talks with the patient about dental anxiety, fears, and phobia and the situations that cause them helps his/her patient control the uneasiness. Sometimes the fears, for children especially, result from tales of older siblings or media about the horrors of the dental office. Allowing the child, or older patient, to observe an easy dental prophylaxis is sometimes all that is needed to dissolve that fear. Sometimes the fear appears after a particularly difficult personal appointment; talking through the scenario that preceded the appointment and how that particular problem is unlikely to arise again may relieve that fear. Occasionally, the only treatment is to provide a mild sedative such as nitrous oxide during the appointment or a pre-treatment sedative such as valium.

Reducing anxiety

Dentists have been using monologue to distract patients for many years. Relaxation techniques such as yoga, meditation, and biofeedback help the patient arrive for the appointment with less anxiety. The dentist seeing the patient on time leaves less time waiting and less time for anxiety to build. Since the advent of portable radios and tape players, patients can choose the music they want to hear through the headphones. Newer hand pieces that make less noise help to reduce anxiety as well. Since much of the anxiety is caused by lack of control of the appointment, anything that helps the patient to feel more in control of what is happening makes the patient more comfortable.

Conscious sedation using nitrous oxide and oxygen is a well-known method for relieving anxiety and increasing relaxation; in addition, it provides some analgesia and decreases the awareness of time and the details of the appointment. The ability to increase a sense of well-being (providing euphoria) is the basis for recreational use and abuse that occurs in some dental offices. Local anesthetics and vasoconstrictors that affect the CNS, the CVS, and the respiratory system are used frequently. The anesthetic blocks the nerve impulses to the brain, and provide the numbness that allows the dentist to work in the area. Local anesthetics are vasodilators and need the counteraction of vasoconstrictors to decrease vasodilation.

The vasoconstrictors keep the anesthetic in the local area as well as restricting blood flow to the area.

Anesthetized patients

Local anesthetics in the proper dosage block nerve impulses to the brain and, at the end of the appointment, disperse without incident. Low levels of local anesthetics have no affect on the CNS or the CVS. Mild sedation and drowsiness, within 5 to 10 minutes of the injection, are the primary signs that the patient is experiencing a toxic reaction to lidocaine. Overdose can cause convulsions, CNS depression, respiratory depression, and respiratory arrest. Overdose of local anesthetics can produce decreased heart contractions and output and rate. Non-overdose levels of local anesthetics can relax the bronchial smooth muscles, but overdose can lead to cardiovascular collapse by massive peripheral vasodilation and to respiratory arrest secondary to CNS depression.

Compromised Patients

An updated medical and dental history is imperative before treatment

Many times a medical impairment is not obvious at first glance. Even when a disability is apparent, the hygienist can only guess at the medications that the patient takes before reading the medical history and reviewing it with the patient and his/her caregiver. Each medicine has particular indications and contraindications for treatment, and each patient has particular needs that must be met if he/she is to receive the best possible dental treatment. Each disabled patient also deserves to be treated with all the dignity of a patient without disability and to be encouraged to provide as much self care as is possible. Only a review of medical and dental history with the patient and his/her caregiver can provide the information necessary for this level of care.

Dental care for patients with medical and physical disabilities

Debralee Nelson defines a disability "as a permanent or long-term condition that limits an individual's ability to perform usual tasks". The classification of a disability should be considered. Is it developmental and limits learning ability or communication? Is it medical and affects major organs of the body? Is it associated with the arms and legs, with paralysis or the loss of limbs? Does it involve sensory perceptions such as hearing or sight? Or is the disability caused by the degeneration of the nervous system or the immune system? After considering which part of the body is affected, the health care worker must consider how well the patient performs the activities of daily living, i.e. how well can the patient take care of him/herself? After considering all these conditions, the health care worker must plan with the patient and his/her caregiver how to provide optimal dental care.

Special needs patients

Geriatric patients have special needs even when they have no physical disabilities. They usually have a list of medications that must be considered before drugs are administered in the dental office. Sometimes the dental health worker must move slowly and explain each element of treatment to prevent overwhelming the patient. Correct positioning of the chair is important for the patient with cardiac or respiratory problems to allow comfortable respiratory function. Pregnant patients need careful chair positioning in order to breathe properly. Patients with eating disorders need instruction detailing care of the mouth and teeth after they vomit. All these patients need instruction regarding preventing or treating dry mouth and gingivitis. These patients should be encouraged to keep regular appointments with primary care physicians as well as dental appointments.

Performing Periodontal Procedures

Etiology and Therapy

Risk factors

Unchanging

One of the unchanging risk factors for periodontal disease is gender. Women, particularly pregnant women, seem to have more hormone fluctuations than men do. Hormone fluctuations associated with puberty also contribute to gingivitis and, if not treated, periodontitis. Genetic structure can predispose a patient to periodontal disease, and congenital deficiencies in the immune system are features that make periodontal disease more likely. Bacterial populations in the oral environment become unbalanced when the immune system is not working efficiently. These factors can be managed through meticulous oral hygiene, but they can not be eliminated completely. There are also conditions, such as diabetes, that contribute to periodontal disease by reducing the efficacy of neutrofil function. A past history of periodontal disease also increases the risk of renewed periodontal disease. These conditions do not change even if periodontal health improves.

Changeable

Poor oral hygiene is the principle factor in gingivitis and periodontal disease. When the patient begins to remove all the plaque and disturb the bacteria in the oral environment daily, gingivitis disappears, and periodontal disease subsides to a manageable level. Age is considered a changing factor because of the fluctuating hormones of puberty, pregnancy, and menopause. Good oral hygiene can prevent gingivitis for these age groups. "Tobacco use is one of the most significant risk factors in development and progression of periodontal disease". Tobacco users exhibit more bone loss, greater pocket depths, and more calculus, even though they have the same or less inflammation and plaque than people who do not use tobacco. Nicotine reduces neutrofil efficacy and changes the blood flow to gingiva causing a decreased immune response.

Nutrition and medications

As in every other health situation, nutrition provides the building blocks to the immune system to repair tissues and block disease. The nutrients associated with wound healing are the most important nutrients for healing and maintaining healthy periodontal tissues. Protein, vitamin C, vitamin A, and zinc promote tissue formation and healing and increase resistance to infection. Folic acid, vitamin B12 and iron improve red blood cell formation, and vitamin K affects clotting time.

In contrast, some medications that are necessary for overall health maintenance seem to increase periodontal problems. The severity of the reaction to meds varies with each patient. Phenytoin, calcium channel blockers, and cyclosporine cause gingival hyperplasia. Hyperplasic gingiva is hard for the patient to clean adequately. Some medications (anorectics, anticholinergics, anticonvulsants, antidepressants, antihistamines, antihypertensives, antiparkinson, antipsychotics, muscle relaxants, and acne treatment) cause xerostomia. Other medications change the host resistance to infection or cause abnormal bleeding.

Plaque and calculus

Plaque provides the sub-structure of bacterial by-products and food debris that attracts the minerals in saliva and sulcular fluid. The precipitated salts, usually calcium compounds, mineralize the plaque making it too hard to remove with floss or toothbrush. Supragingival calculus attaches above the gingival margin. It is usually easily removed by the hygienist. Subgingival calculus is usually brown-black and harder to remove due to the viscosity of the secular fluid and the inaccessibility in the pocket. The calculus has a rough, porous surface and attracts more minerals to grow harder and irritate gingival tissue. Rough restorations, partial dentures, orthodontic appliances and malocclusions are other places that attract plaque and bacteria. Missing and migrating teeth increase bone loss, and mouth breathing dehydrates tissues causing hyperplasia and inflammation.

Influence of systemic disease

Any disorder that the immune system works to repair uses resources that should be reserved to maintain and repair periodontal tissues. Microorganisms flourish, become unbalanced, and destroy periodontal tissues. Ulcerated, damaged periodontal tissues provide points of entry for the microorganisms to enter the blood stream, the circulatory system, and other parts of the body.

Diabetes, especially uncontrolled diabetes, increases the risk of developing periodontal disease by exaggerating the inflammatory response and reducing the ability for wounds to heal. Periodontal disease increases the risks for cardiovascular disease when periodontal pathogens make small clots that can block arteries. Human immunodeficiency virus produces rapid progression of periodontitis which, in turn, leads to further inflammatory response and further immune deficit. Neutrofil disorders increase the progression of periodontal disease because of faulty immune response. Pregnant women with periodontal disease can deliver low birth weight babies because inflammatory toxins affect fetal development.

Mechanisms of bacteria

Bacteria cause damage either by the toxins released as by-products or by initiating exaggerated immune response from the host. Some bacteria invade tissues, and some use enzymes to dissolve connective tissue. Some bacteria use receptor proteins that attach to healthy tissue while others release endotoxins to cause inflammatory response. Aerobic bacteria need oxygen to survive; they are found in areas that are oxygen-rich. Anaerobic bacteria do not need oxygen to survive; they are found deep in the sulcus and other areas that have little or no oxygen supply. Facultative anaerobes can use oxygen, or they can survive without it when necessary. Bacteria are also classified according to their metabolism. Fermentors are gram-positive bacteria that metabolize carbohydrates and ferment the sugars. Nonfermentors use proteins as their food source.

Aerobic bacteria

Immediately after teeth are cleaned, an acellular, organic layer called *pellicle* forms. It provides attachment to the tooth and receptors for bacteria to attach to the tooth.

More bacteria accumulate and become supragingival plaque. As the plaque matures, gram-positive cocci predominate. As more bacteria colonize, facultative anaerobic microorganisms increase and gradually prepare the plaque for anaerobic bacteria. After supragingival plaque matures and more layers of facultative anaerobic bacteria colonize, the plaque grows into the sulcus. Less oxygen is available, so facultative bacteria diminish and Gram-negative anaerobic bacteria dominate. Subgingival plaque is loosely adherent and more toxic than attached plaque. The most significant species of bacteria associated with periodontal disease are *Porphyromonas gingivalis, Actinobacillus actinomycetemcomitans,* and *Prevotella intermedia.*

Addressing gum disease

The hygienist should, first, listen to the patient's complaint. As he/she reviews the medical and dental history with the patient, the hygienist learns about past and present complaints and can calm the patient for the clinical assessment. During the intra-oral exam, the hygienist measures gingival recession and the distance from the CEJ to the base of the pocket. This measurement is the best indicator of periodontal tissue damage. The hygienist looks for and measures any furcation involvement or exposure and tooth mobility. The exam continues with an assessment of the condition of the teeth. The teeth are charted indicating caries, restorations and their status, missing teeth, contact relationships, and wear patterns. All these elements of the intra-oral exam provide a basis for the dental team's analysis and treatment plan.

Necessity of radiographs

Dental radiographs are a picture of the internal structure of the teeth and the bone surrounding the teeth. The dentist and hygienist need full mouth radiographs to see how the teeth fit together as well as apices of each of the teeth and the normal bone structures. Bitewings provide a close-up view of restoration margins and indications of possible carious lesions. Periapical radiographs provide that close-up view of bone and periapical pathology and calcified deposits. After looking at the complete picture, the dental team assesses periodontal health as depicted in the radiographs. They look at normal bone patterns. Height of alveolar bone should be 1 to 2 mm apical to tooth's CEJ. The bone contour should match the contour of the CEJ. Lamina dura should outline the tooth roots and alveolar crest. Periodontal ligament space should look uniform from tooth to tooth, and cancellous bone and trabeculae should be clearly defined.

Abnormal bone patterns

The dentist and hygienist should notice indications of bone destruction. Bone loss is radiographically apparent only when the disease has progressed. Bone loss can be horizontal showing that the alveolar ridge is flat and missing the lamina dura at the top rather than having a white, radiopaque line on the crest. The bone height is reduced, and the distance between the CEJ and the bone is greater than 2 mm. Bone loss can be vertical showing a deep trough at the mesial or distal surface of the tooth between the bone and the tooth root. Advanced furca involvement would depict a radiolucent area between the roots of multirooted teeth. Sometimes the lamina dura looks fuzzy as microorganisms begin destruction.

Treatment planning goals

Treatment plans must be individualized for each patient. The dentist and hygienist must consider the medical and dental history of the patient as well as the patient's attitude regarding his own health and dental needs. The evidence of the intra-oral exam is a major consideration as are the proposed methods for successfully treating each component. Methods for controlling etiologic and predisposing factors are always included in a good treatment plan. Each patient need should be prioritized with emergency situations and painful conditions treated first and progressing to the long-term treatment needs. Patient education (plaque control instruction and review of home oral hygiene results) is an ongoing component in every appointment.

Treatment phases

The phases of treatment and the phases of treatment performed by the hygienist:

- Phase I is the initial therapy and includes patient education, plaque control instruction, informed consent by the patient for treatment, and risk factor counseling. The hygienist scales and root planes and the dentist re-contours margins of restorations.
- Phase II therapy is the surgical treatment which reduces effects of the disease and includes regenerative techniques.
- Phase III therapy is the restorative phase. Phase II and Phase III are sometimes reversed at the dentist's discretion.
- Phase IV is the maintenance phase and continues for the life of the patient. Periodontal disease can be controlled but not cured. The hygienist plays a large part in this supportive phase since the patient needs encouragement to continue doing things that produce good results, and the patient needs some habits, that do not produce good results, fine tuned to produce healthy gingiva without disease.

Oral hygiene aids

Manual tooth brushing after each meal and before bedtime, using one of several techniques, Scrub, roll, Charters, Stillman, modified Stillman, and Bass techniques or a combination of one or more of these techniques is a basic recommendation. Powered toothbrushes are excellent aids for plaque control; it is physically impossible for a human to brush the same number of strokes per minute that a powered brush provides. Dental floss is the best aid to clean between the teeth because it will pass through the contacts down to the sulcus and wrap around the tooth to scrape the plaque off the tooth and disturb microorganisms that are not removed. Floss comes in a large variety of thicknesses, flavors, and a choice of string or floss attached to toothpicks.

Classes of periodontal disease

The classes of periodontal disease as classified by the American Academy of Periodontology:

- *Class I – gingival disease:* Involves inflammation characterized by changes in color, gingival form, position, surface appearance, and presence of bleeding and/or exudates
- *Class II – early periodontitis:* Gingival inflammation progresses deeper into periodontal structures and alveolar bone crest, evidence by slight loss of connective attachment and alveolar bone
- *Class III – moderate periodontitis:* Increased destruction of periodontal structures and noticeable bone loss, possible tooth mobility and furcation involvement
- *Class IV – advanced periodontitis:* Major bone loss usually accompanied by tooth mobility and furcation involvement
- *Class V – refractory periodontitis:* Includes patients with multiple disease sites that continue to demonstrate attachment loss after appropriate therapy – also includes patients with recurrent disease at single or multiple sites; sites continue to be infected by periodontal pathogens no matter how thorough or frequent treatment is provided.

Soft tissue management

There are four objectives of soft tissue management therapy provided by the dental hygienist. The hygienist must remove bacterial plaque and eliminate the etiological conditions that cause disease. He/she should teach the patient how to remove new plaque and microorganisms that develop every day. The patient and the hygienist must keep the plaque off in order to promote repair of periodontal health and prevent recurrence. Removal of toxins, calculus, and other irritants makes the oral environment more favorable for connective tissue reattachment and healing. The improved oral health should slow or stop the progression of periodontal disease, and, if further treatment is necessary, the tissues must be prepared for surgical therapy.

Periodontal debridement removes tooth surface irritants, and is usually the initial step in soft tissue management. Scaling removes plaque and calculus from tooth surfaces using hand-activated instruments or sonic and ultrasonic instruments. Gingival curettage removes the epithelial lining of the periodontal pocket by scraping the surface with a curette or other sharp instrument. Root planing smoothes root surfaces including rough cementum and dentin. SPR combines scaling and root planing. Prophylaxis is the mechanical removal of plaque from teeth. When gingiva is no longer bleeding, coronal polishing removes stains and non-mineralized plaque from tooth crowns with a slow speed handpiece. Selective polishing is used when only a few surfaces of teeth have extrinsic stain. The techniques can be used singly or in combination at the hygienist's discretion during each appointment, but there is progression toward polishing after the gingiva is healthy.

Powered instruments for soft tissue management

EVA Prophylaxis System made by Unitek uses files and points for the removal of overhanging margins of restorations and the interproximal re-contouring of restorations . Sonic scalers that attach to the high-speed hand piece vibrate 2000 to 6000 cycles per second. Ultrasonic scalers can be either magnetostrictive or piezoelectric systems which vibrate between 20,000 to 40,000 cycles per second. These are effective for the removal of calculus and cause less hand stress for the hygienist to use. The new, slimmer tips make instrumentation in narrow pockets easier without distending the gingiva as much as hand-powered instruments. There is a contra-indication for use with patients wearing older pacemakers. Newer pacemakers are usually shielded and are not affected by the electromagnetic field.

Non-surgical therapy

There is documentation that non-surgical therapy is successful in many cases. Improved home oral hygiene is a prominent result of successful patient education and plaque control instruction. Patients express interest in newer and more convenient hygiene aids and occasionally have tips about what works for the hygienist to pass on to other patients. Less bleeding on probing, shallower probing depths, and improved gingival color are readily apparent. Re-attachment occurs in many cases. Continued monitoring at three or four month intervals provides opportunities for the patient, the hygienist, and the dentist to treat any re-occurrences of gingival bleeding before the disease returns to progressive status. In clinics where monitoring of microorganism populations is possible, the dental team finds that there are more aerobic bacteria and fewer anaerobic bacteria.

Antibiotic treatment

The hygienist monitors healing at each phase of soft tissue management therapy. After the initial soft tissue management therapy, the dentist and hygienist sometime decide that healing would progress more rapidly with the addition of antibiotic treatment that targets specific microorganisms. The antibiotic can be delivered locally by placing concentrated tetracycline in the sulcus where it blocks the production of collagenase, or antibiotics can be delivered systemically. *Actinobacillus actinomycetemcomitans* is very susceptible to systemically delivered tetracycline. Metronidazole targets anaerobic Gram-negative bacilli, and when combined with tetracycline, it is useful for treating ANUG and HIV. Penicillin is not effective for periodontal disease because the enzymes produced by periodontal pathogens break down the penicillin. Local delivery of tetracycline embedded fibers

(Actisite), biodegradable chlorhexidine in a gelatin strip (PerioChip), doxycycline gel (Atridox), minocycline powdered microspheres (Arestin), and antimicrobial rinse irrigation have proved to be effective means of reducing microorganisms.

Local delivery of antibiotics

Most states allow the hygienist, under the supervision of the dentist, to place local delivery products in the sulcus of the patient with periodontal disease. Actisite fibers are left in the pocket for ten days and removed. PerioChip is biodegradable in ten days and can be placed in pockets greater than 5 mm. Atridox is injected into the pocket where it conforms to the shape of the pocket and solidifies. It biodegrades in seven days. Arestin is premixed, pre-measured powder microspheres that are injected into the pocket; the microspheres are bioresorbed. Chlorhexidine or other antimicrobial rinses can be injected into the pocket to irrigate and kill microorganisms for twelve hours. Each of these treatments delivers the antimicrobial directly to the diseased site, and each has a low risk for antibacterial resistance.

Subgingival irrigation

Studies show that subgingival irrigation with antimicrobial agents in combination with scaling and root planing provides a greater benefit to the patient than scaling and root planing alone. However, the antimicrobial agent must meet a few criteria. The antimicrobial agent must reach the bottom of the pocket in order to destroy disease-causing anaerobic bacteria. The antimicrobial agent is usually delivered to the bottom of the pocket through a hand syringe with an attached cannula tip. The concentration of antimicrobial agent must be enough to kill the bacteria, and the agent must exhibit substantivity. The most common antimicrobial agents in use at this time are 0.12% chlorhexidine digluconate, 0.4% stannous fluoride, and 0.05% providone-iodine. All of these agents cause staining if used long-term, but none cause prohibitive staining when used as subgingival irrigation agents.

Periodontal surgery

When non-surgical treatment (scaling and root planing) and antibiotics do not produce pockets that are shallow enough to facilitate good oral hygiene at home, periodontal surgery should be considered. Gingival bleeding should have been eliminated, anaerobic microorganisms should have been reduced, and bone loss should have stopped by the time non-surgical and antibiotic treatments have been completed. The hygienist should see the patient for follow-up visits three weeks and six weeks after scaling and root planing treatments to analyze the results of non-surgical treatment. If this treatment is not successful by the criteria established for depth of pockets and gingival appearance, periodontal surgery is probably the best choice for further treatment.

Indications for gingivectomy, gingivoplasty, periodontal flap surgery, mucogingival surgery, and gingival graft procedures

Both gingivectomy and gingivoplasty re-establish a healthy gingival contour by trimming diseased gingiva. A gingivectomy removes fibrous gingiva to provide a shallower pocket, to remove hyperplastic gingiva, and to lengthen a crown so that gingiva does not interfere with restorations or so that restorations do not interfere with gingival health. Gingivoplasty is not intended to eliminate pockets or lengthen crowns. The dentist, or periodontist, performs periodontal flap surgery when he/she needs to expose root or bone surfaces to remove diseased tissue or calculus. Mucogingival surgery creates an environment that encourages attachment of gingiva to the bone. Gingival grafts are sometimes necessary to replace diseased gingiva with healthy gingiva from another location in the mouth or to fill in areas of receded gingiva.

Maintenance appointments

Patients with periodontal disease are usually scheduled for 3-month reassessment and maintenance appointments. Periodontitis can be controlled, but it can not be cured. Even when all visible signs of inflammation have been eliminated, and there is no bleeding on probing, the microbial flora can easily become unbalanced again and the patient can have further bone loss. The periodontal maintenance appointments provide an opportunity to evaluate the periodontium for signs of reoccurring disease. The sulci should be probed for increased pocket depths and evaluated for renewed bleeding. The patient's oral hygiene should be evaluated for efficacy, and when necessary, the patient should be encouraged to improve his/her technique and effectiveness. If the patient can not, or will not, provide good oral hygiene at home and appear for evaluation and periodontal maintenance appointments, there is little value in periodontal therapy.

Compliance is a major problem if the patient does not understand the importance of good oral hygiene at home and regular, frequent maintenance appointments with the hygienist. Instruction presented at the patient's level of understanding with examples to which the patient can relate are a very important part of periodontal therapy. There are times that the patient, especially senior citizens, understands how important maintenance is, but he/she is afraid that the appointment will be as uncomfortable as the initial debridement and scaling appointments were. The hygienist should be thorough in explaining that most of the discomfort of initial appointments was caused by manipulating inflamed tissue. (Removing a sticker from a finger is uncomfortable, but removing it can allow healing and an end to the discomfort.) Sometimes economics or the influence of family and friends weigh more heavily in the decision-making process than the hygienist's instructions and education.

Patient education is the primary technique for improving compliance; however, patient education can be one of the main reasons that patients are noncompliant. If the instruction is too complicated, or too many oral hygiene aids are introduced too quickly, the patient can become confused; he might decide that oral hygiene is too hard to do right, and give up. Therefore, patient education should be simple, uncomplicated, and in the patient's comprehension level (no "big" words unless the patient uses "big" words). The instruction should involve techniques that the patient can perform easily with some practice (Learning to floss is like learning to write one's name – most people can do it, but practice makes it easier).

Dealing with patient claims

What happens if a patient returns to the clinic for a yearly prophy appointment and says that the hygienist did not tell him that he had periodontal disease that was causing bone loss? The first thing that the hygienist should do is to look at clinic notes to confirm that he/she did advise the patient of his periodontal disease and advised him to return in one week to begin scaling and root planing therapy. Clinical notes are a legal document with details of the patient's appointment and the therapy that was performed. Details of the presence or absence of plaque, compliance to instructions and notes concerning progress of healing are helpful in future appointments to provide evidence for completed treatment when non-surgical therapy is not enough to control the disease. . Details of the procedures performed, the instructions given, and any prescriptions and oral hygiene aids given are important parts of the clinical notes.

Plaque index

The most valuable use for a plaque index in the clinic is for patient education. When the hygienist uses a disclosing agent that stains plaque on the teeth, the patient has visible evidence of plaque that he is missing, and in which areas he is missing plaque, when he cleans his teeth. The disclosing solutions that stain plaque with two colors, indicating the length of time that the plaque has been on the patient's teeth, are especially helpful. Recording the score in the patient's chart provides an ongoing record of improvement in oral hygiene. If the hygienist allows the patient to brush off the plaque after it has been stained, the patient learns how long he should be brushing to remove all the plaque.

Periodontal disease recurrence

Recurrence can be because of one or a combination of factors. Insufficient plaque control is the first reason that the hygienist thinks of, but that is usually only part of the reason for recurrence of periodontal disease. Restorations can become cracked, or the tooth around a restoration may crack and allow bacteria to proliferate beyond the reach of good oral hygiene. Systemic conditions can change, putting more stress on the immune system and allowing fewer white blood cells to periodontal sites. Sometimes the patient just needs more frequent maintenance appointments. Whatever the cause, when periodontal disease returns, the therapy begins again. Inflammation must be eliminated, anaerobic microorganisms must be reduced, and conditions must be evaluated for antibiotic or surgical therapy.

Dental implants

Patients with periodontal disease

Good candidates for dental implants must have excellent oral hygiene, fairly good healing ability, adequate bone to hold the implant, and motivation to make the implant procedure successful. An established patient will have a chart with details of dental history and oral hygiene care. If the patient lost his/her teeth because of neglected periodontal disease, chances are that he/she will neglect proper care and maintenance of implants. A medical history will provide information about systemic conditions that might contra-indicate good healing. The dentist, oral surgeon, and prosthodontist will work together to decide if the patient's alveolar bone is adequate to hold an implant, and the dentist's and hygienist's conference with the patient will provide information regarding patient motivation.

Cleaning and maintaining

Maintenance for dental implants should be similar, but different from maintenance for natural teeth. Assessment of tissues, probing implant sulcus depths, evaluating for mobility, assessing and removing plaque and calculus, and obtaining yearly radiographs are necessary for implants just as they are for natural teeth. However, conventional, metal instruments can scratch the titanium surfaces of implants. Plastic instruments are recommended for removing soft and hard deposits and for probing. Sonic and ultra-sonic instruments as well as air polishing are contra-indicated. Selective rubber-cup polishing with tin oxide or polishing with fine-grit commercial paste is acceptable. The bridge supported by the implants should be removed at least yearly to allow for debridement of the implant and to evaluate for stability.

Cleaning implants at home

Each implant system is different and requires the patient to develop techniques that he did not use for cleaning natural teeth in addition to using familiar methods. If the bridge, or prosthesis, is removable, it must be removed daily to clean. The implant that is above the gingival margin should be brushed gently and flossed. Occasional soaking of an overdenture may be necessary. If the prosthesis is not removable, toothbrushes and interproximal cleaning aids with soft, nylon core tips should be used to gently brush all surfaces. Floss, floss threaders, dental tape, wooden and plastic picks, and rubber-tipped stimulators are excellent cleaning aids. Home care methods should be evaluated with the patient at each appointment.

Preventive Agents

Fluoride

Studies have shown that fluoride, when taken systemically in concentrations of 1ppm, reduces decay about 50% – 60%. Fluoride may occur naturally in water; it can be added to drinking water; or it can be taken as a supplement. Greater concentration than 1ppm causes white or brown spots to occur on the developing tooth. If fluoridated water is not available, supplements in liquid drop form, tablets, lozenges, and oral rinses are available. Patients between six months and 14 years of age need fluoride to mineralize developing teeth. Patients with rampant caries, regardless of age, can benefit from fluoride supplements. Elderly patients or patients with gingival recession and exposed root surfaces need fluoride to desensitize and mineralize surfaces. Fluoride is also antibacterial and helpful to reduce the number of microorganisms in the oral environment.

Types of fluoride

Fluoride is usually found in combination with tin, phosphates, or sodium. Stannous fluoride is used in 8% concentration in the dental office. Since the pH is 2.4 to 2.8, stannous fluoride is taken up by the teeth easily. It must be prepared immediately before use due to instability of the formula. SnF is not popular with patients because it tastes bitter and metallic; it also causes extrinsic brown stains and gingival irritation if used long term. Acidulated phosphate fluoride at 1.23% concentration is a combination of 2.0% NaF and 0.34% hydrofluoric acid. Like SnF, it is easily absorbed by teeth due to 3.0 to 3.5 pH. It can cause roughening, pitting or etching of porcelain and composite restorations, but patients usually like the new flavors that are available. Sodium fluoride in 2% concentrations has 9.2 (basic) pH, has an acceptable taste, does not discolor teeth or cause gingival irritation.

The body uses fluoride to make teeth resistant to caries

Most, 86% to 97%, of the fluoride ingested is absorbed in the stomach. As it moves through the circulatory system, fluoride replaces hydroxyapatite crystals in the teeth and bones with fluorapatite, making them harder and more resistant to decay or breakage. The enamel surfaces of the teeth will absorb topical fluoride for several years. Fluoride is deposited first at the dentinoenamel junction. While teeth are developing, excess fluoride can cause hypomineralized spots on the teeth called fluorosis. Skeletal fluorosis can also occur when excess fluoride occurs over a long period of time. Kidney damage can occur when some minerals remain rather than being excreted through the kidneys, sweat glands, and feces.

How fluoride is applied in the dental office

There are several methods for applying fluoride in the dental office. With paint on method the teeth are isolated using cotton rolls or gauze pads to block saliva ducts. With the saliva ejector in one hand, the hygienist dries the teeth, and then paints fluoride on the teeth with a small brush or a cotton-tip applicator. The hygienist keeps all teeth moist with the fluoride gel or liquid. After the recommended time, the patient expectorates excess fluoride. This is the best method for treating a child's teeth with fluoride; the hygienist controls the amount of fluoride and saliva in the mouth to prevent inadvertent swallowing. Trays can be used to soak the teeth in fluoride preparation for the appropriate length of time, or the patient can rinse with fluoride for two minutes. The hygienist instructs the patient not to eat or drink anything for 30 minutes.

Fluoride varnishes

Fluoride varnishes are especially recommended for children because the varnish stays on the teeth for 24 to 48 hours after it is applied. The usual formula is 5% sodium fluoride and usually requires only 0.3 to 0.5 ml of varnish to be applied. With this formula and recommended dosage, the child has only 3 to 6 mg of fluoride exposure. The substantivity of 24 to 48 hours improves the chances that each tooth is saturated for optimal caries prevention. Fluoride varnishes are frequently used to desensitize exposed root surfaces. The fluoride desensitizes tooth surfaces by occluding the microscopic tubules that make up the structure of the tooth. As with children, the fluoride remineralizes the root surface making it physically harder and more resistant to decay.

Acute fluoride toxicity

Acute fluoride toxicity is defined as the rapid intake of an excess (4 to 5 grams) dose of fluoride over a short time. The hygienist is not likely to see acute fluoride toxicity in the clinic, but he/she should know how to recognize and treat mild toxic reactions. Nausea, vomiting, hyper-salivation, abdominal pain, diarrhea, cramping of extremities, bronchospasm, cardiac arrest, ventricular fibrillation, fixed and dilated pupils, and hyperkalemia and hypercalcemia are signs that indicate fluoride toxicity. The urgency of the treatment is in direct relation to the "number of multiples of 5 mg/kg of fluoride ingested". Brian & Cooper recommend induction of vomiting, ingestion of a fluoride-binding agent (e.g. milk, liquid or gel antacids that contain aluminum or magnesium hydroxide), and seeking immediate medical attention.

Fluorsis

Patients are at risk for fluorosis when they ingest water with natural concentrations of fluoride more than 1ppm over long periods, increase intake of food with high levels of fluoride, and consume low calcium diets. Fluorosis is the developmental defect in the tooth enamel that appears as matte white or brown spots on teeth. It is usually symmetrical in the mouth. Questionable to very mild fluorosis looks like small opaque areas on incisal edges or less than 25% of tooth surfaces. Mild fluorosis is characterized by white opacities that involve less than 50% of tooth surfaces. Moderate fluorosis affects all enamel surfaces with frequent brown staining. Teeth with severe fluorosis present discrete pitting and brown stains. Teeth look normal when they erupt, but they pick up posteruptive exogenous stains from the diet.

Sealants

Sealants in the dental office refer to the organic polymer that dentists or hygienists place on the occlusal surfaces of permanent (and sometimes primary) teeth to prevent bacteria from getting into the deep, developmental grooves and fissures of the teeth. Primary teeth, usually, do not have grooves that are too narrow for toothbrush bristles to clean, but the occlusal surfaces of permanent molars do. When they are beyond the reach of toothbrush or floss, the bacteria cause decay. The resin material flows into the fissure and creates a barrier to microorganisms in the oral environment. First molars are usually sealed as soon as possible after eruption because most six-year-olds have not developed the dexterity to brush well, and the fissures in first molars are deep. Sometimes deep developmental pits on the buccal surfaces of first molars are sealed as well.

Some permanent teeth are not sealed

When the grooves of the occlusal surfaces are not deep, there is no need to place sealants there. Teeth that have restoration of occlusal surfaces are not sealed. Carious lesions are not sealed. A patient who can not control his/her tongue well enough for the hygienist and assistant to keep a dry field is not a good candidate for sealants since sealant material can be placed only on a dry tooth. A partially erupted tooth that has one fossa that can be isolated and dried can have sealant material placed in that fossa. Incipient lesions can be sealed at the discretion of the dentist. If the surface has no deep pits or fissures, or if the tooth can not be isolated and completely dried, sealant material can not be applied successfully.

Procedure for cleaning and etching a tooth prior to placing sealant material

The teeth are thoroughly cleaned of all plaque and debris. The tooth is isolated with cotton rolls, a rubber dam, or cheek triangles and dried with the air syringe. The tooth must be completely dry to avoid diluting the etching gel. High volume evacuation used by an assistant improves chances of keeping the tooth dry and the etching material and the sealant material from touching gingiva or the tongue. The acid etch creates micropores in the tooth surface to allow mechanical retention of the resin material. It also removes contamination and bacteria from the enamel. The phosphoric acid (15% - 50%) in liquid or gel form stays on the tooth for 15 to

60 seconds according to manufacturer's instructions. The etching material is thoroughly washed off, and the tooth is dried again. The occlusal surface of the tooth should look chalky.

Placement of the resin

According to manufacturer's directions, a small amount of resin is allowed to flow into pits and fissures. Care should be taken not to place resin on cusp tips or margins and to avoid overfilling to a high, flat surface. Resin that must be cured with a light requires that the patient, the hygienist, and the assistant wear protection from the ultraviolet or visible blue light. The light should cover the entire tooth (about 2 mm away from the surface) for 20 to 30 seconds as recommended by the manufacturer. Self-curing resin requires that the hygienist mix the monomer and catalyst before placing it on the prepared tooth. It takes about 2 to 3 minutes to harden. After the resin is cured, the hygienist should use an explorer to check for defects. Articulating paper helps to locate high spots that need adjusting.

Oral rinses

Oral rinses reduce the numbers of microorganisms, and improve odor of the mouth and decrease the risk for caries and periodontal disease. Oxygenating agents, such as hydrogen peroxide, clean by bubbling bacteria away and work only as long as the bubbles last. Over use can cause an imbalance of oral flora and black hairy tongue. Chlorhexidine gluconate (0.12%) is a prescription rinse that causes cell wall lysis of Gram-positive and –negative bacteria and fungi. It is time-released for about 12 to 24 hours. Essential oils, such as Listerine, are used to reduce plaque and gingivitis. The original formula contains 26.9% alcohol, but newer formulas have only 21.6% alcohol. "Quaternary ammonia compounds decrease bacterial cell wall permeability and metabolism, posses no substantivity, and are recommended for halitosis, not gingivitis". Sanguinarine and stannous fluoride change bacterial cell walls, and alters bacterial cell metabolism and adhesion.

Providing Supportive Treatment Services

Dental Materials

Agencies providing guidelines

The agencies providing guidelines for material performance:

- Food and Drug Administration regulates safety and efficacy of medical and dental materials and devices.
- American Dental Association Council on Scientific Affairs provides a certification (which is not necessary) program. ADA Seal Acceptance Program provides assurance that materials perform as they are advertised. ADA Specification Program provides guidelines for the manufacture of dental materials.
- International Standards Organizations and Federation Dentaire Internationale provide guidelines for international standards.
- Occupational Safety and Health Administration provides safety guidelines for the employees in the workplace.
- ADA Regulatory Compliance Manual provides guidelines for management of waste and other issues within the community at large.
- Materials Safety Data Sheet, published by the manufacturer, provides instructions for safely using, storing, and disposing of material. There should be one sheet for each product used in the dental office.

Dental restorations

Direct restorations are made in the mouth while the patient is in the chair. Indirect restorations are made in a lab using a cast of the structure being restored. Inlays are made to fill teeth using casts of the teeth after caries has been removed and the teeth are prepared for impressions. Crowns and onlays cover the outside of the tooth structure. All of these restorations are cemented to the prepared tooth. Fixed partial dentures (bridges) replace one or more missing teeth. They are cemented to teeth on each side of the missing teeth or to implants. Removable partial dentures are like fixed partial dentures but are attached with clasps rather than being permanently fixed to adjacent teeth. Complete dentures replace the teeth in an endentulous arch.

Most dental restorations are held in place by a mechanical bond. For example, an amalgam filling is stays in the tooth because the dentist removed the carious material and drilled a mushroom-shaped receptacle before packing the amalgam in the tooth. After it hardens, the narrower opening holds the amalgam in place. Resin restorations usually have an epoxy that causes adhesion (unlike molecules attach to one another, i.e. resin to enamel) or cohesion (like molecules attach to one another, welding and direct gold restorations). Zinc polycarboxylate cement and glass ionomer cements demonstrate primary molecular interaction. The most common type of molecular interaction involves physical forces with no chemistry involved. Wetting is another method by which restorations are retained. The adhesive wets the adherend, forming a contact angle close to 0.

<u>Other properties considered</u>

Ductility and malleability must be considered; the material must be able to hold its shape under tension. Flow and creep are important considerations for material that must continually change under load. The material must be hard enough to resist penetration and resist abrasion. Some of the material must thin and flow during working then set to a prescribed shape for the finished product. The ability or inability of the material to conduct heat must be considered as it is placed in certain areas of the mouth. Color changes can enhance or destroy the cosmetic appearance of a restoration. Materials are also chosen by their ability to solidify by cooling or drying with no chemical reaction, and by the ability to solidify by forming a new chemical bond within the structure.

Stress versus strain

Stress is the internal force developed within an object when force is applied from the outside (Stress = Force/Area; lb/in squared). Strain denotes a change in shape caused by a given stress. Compressive stress occurs during compression of the object. Tensile stress is caused by stretching the object. Shear stress happens when one part of the object is forced to slide by the other. Complex stresses and strains are a combination of compressive, tensile, and shear stress. Torsion (twisting), flexion (bending around a midpoint), and diametral tensile (stretching from the diameter) are examples of complex stresses and strains. "Elastic strain disappears when stress is removed" according to Brian & Cooper.

Temporary restorations

Many times a temporary restoration is necessary to protect a tooth that is waiting for a crown. If the dentist is unsure whether the nerve of the tooth with a deep restoration will heal, he might place a medicated temporary restoration. Acrylics similar to denture bases are used when a temporary restoration must look like a natural tooth. Stainless steel or aluminum crowns are frequently used on primary teeth or on permanent molars. These crowns are strong enough for the occlusal forces and easily removed when a permanent restoration is ready. Composite material has an intermediate strength with light flexibility. ZOE (zinc oxide eugenol) provides relief from mild discomfort and reduces inflammation while a healthy nerve recovers.

Tooth-colored permanent restorations

Ceramic restorations are a combination of metal oxides and minerals. They might be glass, concrete, fine crystal, or gypsum. Glass might reinforce dental composites to make them stronger or coat veneers or metallic restorations to make them more appealing. Porcelain used in dentistry is especially formulated. It emits light when illuminated and looks very natural. It is used for denture teeth, crowns and bridgework, veneers, and inlays. Composites are used in class III, IV, and V restorations, to fill spaces of diastemas, and as veneers to cover stained teeth. Enamel and dentin adhesives provide the attachment of restorations to the teeth. These are usually unfilled resins that rely on mechanical attachment of the resin to acid-etched enamel and dentin.

Amalgam

Amalgam is an alloy of two or more metals. Mercury makes the amalgam malleable enough to place in a tooth cavity and silver increases setting expansion and strength. Tin makes the compound mix more thoroughly and adds strength. Tin decreases setting expansion. Copper increases strength, hardness, and the setting expansion. Zinc is frequently added to minimize oxidation. Amalgam is very strong, especially during compression, so an amalgam restoration can remain intact during the heavy crushing force of eating. It is stiff and holds the shape designed by the dentist during the packing of the preparation. As the amalgam is condensed, excess mercury is removed, and the restoration becomes stronger and experiences less dimensional change during setting. The bonding of amalgam to the tooth increases fracture resistance, increases strength, and allows a more conservative preparation.

Polishing

Indications for polishing teeth as a part of routine prophy

Most extrinsic stains can be removed; the amount of stain and the type of stain should be considered when the polishing paste is chosen. Heavier stain requires a coarser paste; light stain requires fine paste. Patients expect polishing as a part of the cleaning process. Many patients consider that their teeth have not been cleaned until the polishing procedure has been finished. Polishing can remove small amounts of loose plaque. Heavy plaque or plaque that has been on teeth more than one day is very difficult to remove with a polishing cup; using a curette is preferred. Polishing gives teeth the "squeaky clean" surface that readily accepts etching gel preparatory to application of sealants.

Contraindications for polishing

Soft areas of teeth can be scratched or removed if the polishing procedure is vigorous or if the paste is too coarse. The paste can scratch gold, porcelain, composite, and other aesthetic restorations. Polishing paste is contraindicated for titanium implants; the porcelain crown can be hand-polished with very fine paste to remove stain. Polishing can cause frictional heat and damage primary teeth or other teeth with large pulp chambers. Limiting the speed of the rotating cup and the pressure and amount of time that the cup touches the tooth is recommended. A bacteremia can be initiated from polishing paste entering inflamed gingiva. Aerosols created by rotary instruments carry microorganisms that can enter the unprotected eyes of patients and the respiratory track of patients with infectious disease, immunosuppression and respiratory illness. Using air-polishing instruments with sodium bicarbonate powder is contraindicated for patients on sodium controlled diets.

Methods of polishing

The Porte polisher is a manual device made of a stainless steel handle with a contra-angled end that holds a wooden polishing point. This polisher is safe to use with children and on tooth surfaces that can easily be damaged by the rotating speed of even the slow speed prophy angle. The rubber cup or brush attached to a prophy angle on the slow speed hand piece is the most widely used polishing device. It removes heavy extrinsic stain quickly and efficiently. The air polisher system uses sodium bicarbonate slurry under pressure to remove heavy stain efficiently. The shorter time means less stress on the hand and wrist of the operator. It works better than rubber cup polishing to prepare teeth for the application of pit and fissure sealants.

Impressions and study casts

Rationale for using impression and replication materials

Many restorations can not be fabricated in the mouth, but the lab tech needs an exact replica of the mouth to create the restoration. Impression materials provide the capability to send the necessary portion of the mouth to the lab tech. The impressions record a negative of hard and soft tissues that can be used by the lab tech to construct restorations to replace missing teeth, to construct orthodontic appliances, or for trays used to prevent damage to teeth during sports or sleep. The inelastic materials are rigid and provide an excellent material to mount casts on articulators. Aqueous elastomeric materials (hydrocolloid) include irreversible hydrocolloid (alginate) and reversible hydrocolloid (agar).

Most used impression materials

Impression plaster is used most often as a base to mount study casts on an articulator. ZOE is used for medicated filling material and periodontal surgery dressings. Alginate is used to make a negative of tooth structure to which a restoration is to be attached. Agar gives a highly accurate impression. Both alginate and agar impressions must be poured promptly to avoid dimensional changes. Polysulfide, silicone rubber, and polyvinylsiloxane give excellent detail. Polyvinylsiloxane has the least dimensional change and causes less tissue reaction that polysilfide and silicone rubber. Polyether has the shortest working time and dimension change between polysulfides and silicones. These materials have various working times and must be used according to manufacturer's directions.

Impression versus replication materials

Impression plaster and stone are examples of replication materials used to make a positive reproduction. These materials are mixed and poured into the impression negatives created from the patient's mouth. Plaster is made by heating gypsum at atmospheric pressure; it is porous and irregularly shaped material that is good for attaching study models to articulators. Dental stone is a finer, less porous product made by heating gypsum under steam pressure. The material is good for making the base of study models. Die stone, made by dehydrating gypsum in calcium chloride, is the best product to use for making individual teeth on a model and for making molds for crowns and inlays.

Uses for study casts

Study casts provide documentation of the conditions of the mouth at the beginning of treatment and of progress as it occurs. Study casts are useful in forensic cases. Casts allow the dental team to study the patient's mouth from all angles and to study relationships of the arches to each other and individual teeth. The dental team can see the results of various methods of restoration before a final choice for restoration is made. The dentist can see wear facets, open contacts, rotated teeth, and gingival recession on models. Study models are good educational tools that the dentist or hygienist can show to the patient and demonstrate the best oral hygiene techniques. The patient can practice new techniques on models before going home.

Community Health/Research Principles

Dental hygiene regulating body

Dental hygiene practice is regulated by the American Dental Association, and hygienists work under the supervision of a dentist. Different states have different rules about how closely the dentist supervises the hygienist. The state board of dental examiners in each state controls the clinical requirements for licensure – usually choosing to send candidates to one of the regional boards for clinical exams.

They are Central Regional Dental Testing Service, Northeast Regional Board of Dental Examiners, Southern Regional Testing Agency, and Western Regional Examining Board. The Joint Commission on National Dental Examinations conducts written exams each year to test candidates on academic knowledge. Each state tests candidates regarding ethics and laws of the state in which the candidate wishes to practice.

Public with private practice

Procedures followed in public dental health are very similar to those followed in private practice except that the patient is the community or a group rather than a single person. The private hygienist collects information regarding health and dental history and examines the patient for conditions that need to be corrected. The public hygienist collects information from a survey and analyses it for conditions that need to be corrected (needs assessment). The private practice hygienist plans and implements treatment. The public hygienist plans and implements programs that correct the need of the community. The private hygienist details treatment so that the office personnel can collect payment from the patient or his/her insurance. The public hygienist details needs of the community (the patient) and presents the report to sponsors for funding (before treatment is given). The results of treatment are evaluated for the private patient or the community.

Governmental levels

Four governmental levels of dental public health

- *International – World Health Organization (WHO):* Works to support programs in underdeveloped nations to improve or maintain health with minimal equipment. WHO establishes guidelines for primary healthcare and tracks efficacy of programs internationally.
- *Federal – Department of Health and Human Services (DHHS):* Funds research and acts on oral health problems of national significance.
- *State:* Each state provides consultation services to local departments and administers programs in rural areas not covered by city services. The state governments fund some prevention programs from their Maternal and Child Health Services funds.
- *Local:* Local governments provide direct services at county and city level and initiate dental health legislation such as fluoridation. City and county governments work to provide services to communities within the shrinking availability of federal funds.

Need and demand

The *need* for dental services is a specific oral health problem recognized in the community. The *normative need* is the professionally perceived need regarding the amount of dental services required by the community to become orally healthy. The *perceived need* is the need for dental services that the public believes are necessary for the community to be orally healthy. It refers to the need recognized by the individual in the community. *Demand* occurs when individuals in the community actively seek dental services after learning of the conditions that the dental professional perceives as need. *Use of services* indicates the proportion of the community who seek professional dental treatment within a specific period of time.

Factors affecting service use

The individual who uses dental services most regularly in the United States is a "white, college-educated woman with a higher than average income, who lives in a suburban area, has dental insurance, and possesses the characteristics of good general and oral health". Age is one factor that affects use of dental treatment; as the general population ages, use of dental services by the elderly will increase. Dental services are used least by preschoolers and most by teenagers. More females use dental services than males. Socioeconomic status affects use of dental services; people near or below poverty level without dental insurance use dental services least. Ethnicity seems to affect dental services use; race and ethnicity seem to be related to socioeconomic status, cultural values, and geographic location, so differentiating which affects dental services use most is difficult.

Ideal public health program

The ideal public dental health program should be designed to correct a widespread condition that can, or does, cause morbidity (relative incidence of disease) or mortality (loss of teeth). This program should be easy to learn and dentally and medically safe for all users. It should be inexpensive, affordable and available for most individuals regardless of socioeconomic status, education, income, race, age, or gender. It should not require dental professionals to administer it efficiently. It should be accepted as a solution to individual problems by most patients and should require minimum compliance to be effective. Most importantly, the ideal program should be a valid method of controlling the incidence of the target disease.

Establishing community programs

The first step for planning and implementing a community health problem is to identify the problem. There are various methods of evaluating the population to learn health status, demographics, socioeconomic status, and availability of funding, availability of facilities, availability of manpower, and the status of any presently ongoing programs. After data has been collected for needs assessment and availability of resources, the needs must be prioritized according to primary health problems and the target group with the greatest need. Setting broad goals and narrowing those goals to specific objectives are the next necessary step. Frequently planners devise more than one method for meeting the needs of the population. Following the strategies for implementation and conducting the project are next. Evaluation of the efficacy of the program, during the project and after it has been fully implemented provides information needed to decide to continue the project.

Programs benefit community

Dental health programs for the community seem to bridge the gap between the individuals who qualify for state and federal assistance and those who have dental insurance. Health care costs, especially dental health care costs, have risen while the dental insurance benefits have decreased. The government's contributions to dental care have remained the same without regard to increasing cost of living indices. Community health care administrators have to be more creative when seeking funding for health programs. They look for professional volunteers to provide services and donations of supplies. Local components of dental associations assess the need for services and sponsor programs for their communities to provide for those needs.

Local dental associations

Local components of dental and dental hygiene associations frequently join forces to provide dental screening and preventative care to children in a community. A day is chosen for volunteers to meet with families at a particular place. Dentists screen the children for problems and send those needing dental cleaning and sealants to the hygienists for care. Dental professionals volunteer their time and skills, and dental supply companies frequently donate supplies. Some administrative skills and money for supplies are donated by concerned citizens of the community. Some states have a day designated as sealant day as part of the observance of Dental Health Month or Dental Health Week. Local practices frequently send dental health care workers to schools during Dental Health Month to provide education and samples of supplies to first and second grade students.

Capitation plans

Capitation plans are contracts between providing dentists and insurance companies. The dentist agrees to treat all the patients assigned to him/her by that company for a specific payment based on the number of patients assigned. The dentist receives that same payment each month regardless of the number of assigned patients that are treated that month. There is understanding by the dentist and the insurance company that some patients will need a significant amount of care while others assigned to him/her will require no care that month. The patients receive all the benefits detailed by the company and pay a small amount (called co-pay) established by a schedule in the contract.

Dental service corporations

Dental service corporations originated in 1954 when a trade union joined a district dental society to provide services to children less than 14 years of age. Since that time other not-for-profit corporations have been formed to negotiate and provide dental care contracts. The corporations are governed by the insurance laws of the state in which they are incorporated. The private dental practices sign contracts to provide care at group practice rates according to an established fee structure. A committee of nonparticipating dentists conducts post-treatment evaluations to ensure acceptable quality. Indemnity plans are commercial insurance plans that operate for profit. The fees are based on fees most often charged in the area. Direct reimbursement plans require the patient to pay the dentist for care and submit a record of treatment to his/her employer who reimburses the patient. These plans were designed at the community level and have grown to state or nationwide acceptance.

Managed care

Health maintenance organizations (HMOs) were developed in 1973 to lower the cost of health care by dictating specific cost for specific procedures. They have reduced health care costs by increasing ambulatory care procedures. Dental maintenance organizations usually charge a separate premium for coverage. There seems to be no difference between DMO and prepaid group fee schedules. Preferred provider organizations (PPOs) offer a contract between the provider and the organization for a predetermined fee schedule. PPO groups allow the patient to choose from a list of preferred providers who charge a lower than average fee for procedures. Managed care organizations allow patients to choose practitioners whom they like. Public financing by federal, state, and tribal governments provide health and dental care for groups such as the military, Native Americans, and penitentiary inmates.

Federal government programs

The Maternal and Child Health Services provide health and dental care for infants and children through WIC and Head Start programs. Medicaid, since 1965, is a joint federal and state program that provides oral health care for individuals less than 21 years of age. Medicare provides insurance protection for disabled individuals or those 65 years of age and older, but this program excludes dental care. Medicare will pay for oral/maxillofacial problems that relate to a medical condition. The National Health Service Corps deploys commissioned officers and civil service employees to areas that are underserved by health care workers. State Health Agencies provide preventative and emergency dental care to children less than 18 years of age. They provide limited restorative care.

Limiting managed care organizations

The simple answer is that managed care organizations of all kinds pay less for any procedure than private insurance or patients who pay cash. The fee schedules are set to reimburse the practice for cost of supplies and overhead with very little compensation for the dentists or hygienist's skills and time. Some dental practices try to see more patients per day to offset the lower fees. Other practices add more patients to the assignment list and hope that very few of them require major work. Some practices limit the number of managed care patients that are seen each day and schedule major work for private insurance patients to balance the income.

Scientific Information/Results

Considering scientific information

Since the community is the patient, and the dental health provider can not properly care for his/her patient without knowing what that patient needs, the hygienist must collect and analyze information about the patient. The information about the patient must be collected in a manner that can be duplicated. Following scientific collection protocol is the only way that information about a large group can be verified and validated. When he/she analyzes the information collected, the hygienist can see areas of concern that are common to a majority of the individuals in the community. The community is the patient, and treatment is chosen to benefit the community, but individuals are considered as well.

Factors affecting community health

The health of the community is affected by host concerns such as age, gender, race, and immune system efficacy. A community with an average age of 60 years has different concerns than the community with an average age of 30 years. The amount of sun exposure the individual has, the pollutants in the air and water, and presence of radiation (if any) affect the health of an individual and, therefore, the community. A community located near the equator with direct sunlight all year has more concerns about the damages of radiation from the sun than the community in Norway or Alaska. Lifestyle considerations such as education, socioeconomic status and cultural mores, drug and alcohol consumption, and diet have a dynamic affect on individuals and communities.

Descriptive versus experimental studies

Descriptive studies are concerned more with the characteristics of a disease rather than trying to determine a cause for the disease. The incidence study describes the number of new cases of the disease within a specific time period. The prevalence study describes the total number of cases at a particular point in time or within a particular period of time. Descriptive studies are designed to increase understanding of a disease and to plan and evaluate healthcare studies that prevent or control the disease.

Experimental studies are designed to establish a cause for the disease. The study usually involves manipulating independent variables and dependent variables in one group while monitoring a control group. Comparisons are made to test a hypothesis that a particular agent alters the natural history of the disease being studied.

Epidemiology studies

Analytical studies are descriptive studies designed to analyze the relationship between and among variables. Longitudinal studies can be descriptive or experimental; they provide observations over a long period of time. Prospective studies are longitudinal studies of subjects over time to determine if a condition develops. Retrospective studies are descriptive studies that investigate previously collected data. Developmental studies examine progression or development of a condition over a period of time using longitudinal approach. Developmental studies are further divided into cohort study which follows one group over time to observe development of a condition. Case history compares a group with a disease to determine factors that relate to its occurrence. Cross-sectional studies observe a group at a point in time to determine occurrence of condition and relate this to other variables in the population.

Internal validity describes how much the change in independent variables influenced the change in the dependent variables. External validity describes the degree to which results can be generalized to community. Validity includes sensitivity -- it tests positive if the condition is present -- specificity – it tests negative if condition is absent and predictive value – identifies presence or absence of condition. The measure must be reliable – can be duplicated by same examiner or a different examiner. The sample size can be determined at random, in stratified random manner, as a systematic sample, or by convenience, which is the least reliable type of sample. Groups should be assigned randomly, without bias. The methods for measuring disease – count (not useful), prevalence, incidence, or using indices – are also important.

Example: How a community dental health worker would use results from a research project in Sweden that studied the effect of diet on dental decay in humans.

The hygienist first should examine the object of the research. Could the consumption of sugar cause dental decay in the patients in this particular practice? The subjects are comparable to the patients in the hygienist's practice, and the hypothesis is logical (sugar turns to acid during the pre-digestion phase). If he/she sees a patient with rampant decay, the hygienist can ask specific questions regarding the patient's diet and recite results of the research regarding sugar in the diet. When he/she correlates the patient's diet with a diet high in carbohydrates, especially refined carbohydrates, the hygienist can teach the patient that cleaning the teeth immediately after eating refined carbohydrates reduces the risk of decay.

Example: How the hygienist would use research results from a study, by the local dental hygiene association, of second grade children and their brushing and flossing habits and the prevalence of decay at the time of the study.

The hygienist could examine results and discuss implementing a program in which individual dental hygiene volunteers arrange visits to local schools to present educational information to the first and second grade students. The students would learn why they need to brush after every meal and brush and floss before bed. By including the first grade students, the student's awareness of the reason for tooth decay is encouraged at a time when they are very impressionable and they want to be more independent. The students would learn how to brush efficiently and that flossing is a learned skill that they can accomplish. Children, like adults, like to learn and apply new skills. Frequent reinforcement of good oral hygiene skills results in fewer teeth lost from decay.

Example: The local dental hygienists association conducted a study of local retirement centers in which the residents were ambulatory and cared for their personal hygiene duties. The hygienists can promote quality care for these senior citizens.

Although it indicated that the residents were responsible for their personal hygiene duties, the study conducted by the dental hygienists association revealed that many of the residents had difficulty holding regular toothbrushes and floss long enough to properly brush and floss their teeth. The hygiene association members could provide powered toothbrushes for more effective brushing in a shorter amount of time, or the members could provide tennis balls, bicycle handlebar grips, or other items to modify the handles of the toothbrushes the residents use. Floss picks and floss holders make flossing easier by extending the reach of the resident into his/her mouth. The residents, like people everywhere, would benefit from regularly scheduled group oral hygiene lessons. Individualized, one on one oral hygiene lessons in which the hygienist watches the resident clean his/her teeth, then "fine tunes" the technique would be especially helpful.

Sample scenarios

Sample Scenario 1

Ms Jones, a member of her local dental hygiene association, has recently volunteered to provide preventive dental services under the supervision of her boss, Dr. Scott, for the residents in Garden Terrace Nursing Home. Prior to her first visit, Ms Jones and her assistant, Mary, set objectives for the dental health program at Garden Terrace. At her initial visit, Ms Jones and Mary document that 15 of the 50 patients assigned to her are edentulous; 3 patients are missing only their third molars; 15 patients are missing 6 or less teeth, and the remaining 18 patients have more than 6 teeth missing. They also documented the number of decayed and filled teeth. Ms Jones and her assistant performed and documented the results of a plaque index and PSR scores. They found that 90% of the 50 patients assigned to them had plaque index scores of 60% or more, and 75% of the 50 patients had PSR scores greater that 2 in two or more quadrants. Ms Jones and Mary then planned how they could meet the needs of their patients within the parameters identified by the dental and hygiene associations.

Which type of epidemiological study Ms Jones and Mary conduct?

A. Analytical
B. Descriptive
C. Prospective
D. Experimental
E. Cross-sectional

B. Descriptive – Ms Jones and Mary conducted descriptive studies of the fifty geriatric patients assigned to them. This study is designed to describe the conditions present within the population. They also documented the health concerns of the assigned patients. The descriptions documented reveal information that allows Ms Jones and Mary to formulate a plan to meet the needs of the population. They can present their assessment and plan for implementation to Dr. Scott for his approval before collecting resources. They can also report their findings to their hygiene association for comparison with the results of studies performed by other volunteer hygienists at Garden Terrace and other nursing homes. The combined reports of all the hygienists provide a picture of the general dental health of the elderly patients in the area nursing homes.

Sample Scenario 2

Ms Jones, a member of her local dental hygiene association, has recently volunteered to provide preventive dental services under the supervision of her boss, Dr. Scott, for the residents in Garden Terrace Nursing Home. Prior to her first visit, Ms Jones and her assistant, Mary, set objectives for the dental health program at Garden Terrace. At her initial visit, Ms Jones and Mary document that 15 of the 50 patients assigned to her are edentulous; 3 patients are missing only their third molars; 15 patients are missing 6 or less teeth, and the remaining 18 patients have more than 6 teeth missing. They also documented the number of decayed and filled teeth. Ms Jones and her assistant performed and documented the results of a plaque index and PSR scores. They found that 90% of the 50 patients assigned to them had plaque index scores of 60% or more, and 75% of the 50 patients had PSR scores greater than 2 in two or more quadrants.

What is the significance of the number of missing teeth and which factor influenced the dental health most in this geriatric population?

A. Age
B. Cultural habits
C. Environment
D. Education
E. All of the above

E. All of the above – The total number of missing teeth in this population combined with the number of decayed and filled teeth indicates the prevalence of dental care for this population through the years. The hygienists can consider the age of the patients and recall that most of these patients did not live in areas with fluoridated water supply. Studies have shown that patients who lived in areas with naturally fluoridated water had fewer cavities and fewer teeth lost to decay. The availability of professional dental care in rural areas also influenced the prevalence of decayed teeth, and the quality of dental restorations affected the willingness of patients to have teeth restored rather than extracted. The lack of information available to the public about periodontal disease affected the number of teeth lost to periodontal disease.

Sample Scenario 3

Ms Jones, a member of her local dental hygiene association, has recently volunteered to provide preventive dental services under the supervision of her boss, Dr. Scott, for the residents in Garden Terrace Nursing Home. Prior to her first visit, Ms Jones and her assistant, Mary, set objectives for the dental health program at Garden Terrace. At her initial visit, Ms Jones and Mary document that 15 of the 50 patients assigned to her are edentulous; 3 patients are missing only their third molars; 15 patients are missing 6 or less teeth, and the remaining 18 patients have more than 6 teeth missing. They also documented the number of decayed and filled teeth. Ms Jones and her assistant performed and documented the results of a plaque index and PSR scores. They found that 90% of the 50 patients assigned to them had plaque index scores of 60% or more, and 75% of the 50 patients had PSR scores greater that 2 in two or more quadrants.

What were the objectives that Ms Jones and Mary probably assigned to their program and which has first priority?

A. Control plaque accumulations
B. Control the incidence of periodontal disease
C. Teach residents and nursing aides to de-plaque
D. Arrange for periodic preventive screening
E. Evaluate resident's manual dexterity

E. Evaluate resident's manual dexterity – Evaluating resident's manual dexterity is probably the first objective since Ms Jones and Mary can not plan education seminars for residents and nursing aides until abilities are known. Some of the residents can clean their own teeth, and some residents need help from the aides. However, providing specialized toothbrushes might be all the help that some residents need. A bicycle handlebar grip firmly attached to the toothbrush handle provides a larger, broader handle for an arthritic hand to grasp. A tennis ball at the end of the toothbrush handle does the same. Powered toothbrushes make cleaning teeth more efficient for the resident and for the aide. There are various holders that make flossing easier. Providing preventive screening and regularly scheduled education keeps the goal of clean teeth and healthy gingiva near the front of everyone's mind.

<u>Sample Scenario 4</u>

Ms Jones, a member of her local dental hygiene association, has recently volunteered to provide preventive dental services under the supervision of her boss, Dr. Scott, for the residents in Garden Terrace Nursing Home. Prior to her first visit, Ms Jones and her assistant, Mary, set objectives for the dental health program at Garden Terrace. At her initial visit, Ms Jones and Mary document that 15 of the 50 patients assigned to her are edentulous; 3 patients are missing only their third molars; 15 patients are missing 6 or less teeth, and the remaining 18 patients have more than 6 teeth missing. They also documented the number of decayed and filled teeth. Ms Jones and her assistant performed and documented the results of a plaque index and PSR scores. They found that 90% of the 50 patients assigned to them had plaque index scores of 60% or more, and 75% of the 50 patients had PSR scores greater that 2 in two or more quadrants.

What are the types of resources available for Ms Jones and Mary to meet the objectives of their geriatric dental health program?

A. Willing residents
B. Helpful nursing aides
C. Families of residents
D. Supplies from dental supply companies
E. Mentors from the dental association
F. All of the above

F. All of the above – The residents who are physically and mentally able to clean their own teeth are usually eager to do what they can to keep their mouths healthy. With the help of toothbrushes and floss equipment designed specifically for their particular handicap, they can handle most oral hygiene chores daily. Nursing aides at residential centers have varying amounts of time available to help with oral hygiene chores, but most can help residents who need help with oral hygiene chores. Families of the residents are usually eager to help their loved ones within the time that they have available. Many dental supply companies will donate supplies when they see the need. Most dentists are willing to provide ideas to solve unusual dexterity problems.

Sample Scenario 5

Prior to her first visit, Ms Jones and her assistant, Mary, set objectives for the dental health program at Garden Terrace. At her initial visit, Ms Jones and Mary document that 15 of the 50 patients assigned to her are edentulous; 3 patients are missing only their third molars; 15 patients are missing 6 or less teeth, and the remaining 18 patients have more than 6 teeth missing. They also documented the number of decayed and filled teeth. Ms Jones and her assistant performed and documented the results of a plaque index and PSR scores. They found that 90% of the 50 patients assigned to them had plaque index scores of 60% or more, and 75% of the 50 patients had PSR scores greater that 2 in two or more quadrants. Explain how Ms Jones and Mary would use PSR scores, and the objectives that they probably assigned to their program, as well as which has first priority.

A. To identify the need for restorations
B. To explain to the residents why they need to brush better
C. To identify residents who need follow-up visits with the dentist for complete periodontal testing
D. To identify residents who need more help from their families

C. To identify residents who need follow-up visits with the dentist for complete periodontal testing – PSR is the acronym for Periodontal Screening Recording. The PSR system provides a unified standard for evaluating the periodontal health of patients by evaluating the depth of the sulcus and the absence or presence of bleeding. The PSR is easily done and quickly reveals the need for complete periodontal testing when it is necessary. The hygienist uses a probe with a green band from the 3.5 to 5.5 mm mark. When the green band is visible, the hygienist continues with the probing at the next sextant. When only the red bands are visible, the hygienist stops probing and schedules the patient for a complete periodontal evaluation. The PSR codes do not correlate to any periodontal diagnosis, but the codes do reveal oral conditions to practitioners who are familiar with their meaning.

Special Report- Study Guides and Practice Tests Are Worth Your Time

We believe the following practice tests and guide present uncommon value to our customers who wish to "really study" for the NBDHE tests. While our manual teaches some valuable tricks and tips that no one else covers, learning the basic coursework tested on the exam is also necessary.

Practice Tests

Appleton and Lange's Review for the Dental Hygiene National Board Examination

http://www.amazon.com/exec/obidos/tg/detail/-/083850230X/qid=1089297271/sr=8-9/ref=sr_8_xs_ap_i9_xgl14/104-7475717-5520728?v=glance&s=books&n=507846

Study Guides

Saunders Review of Dental Hygiene

http://www.amazon.com/exec/obidos/tg/detail/-/072167576X/qid=1089297271/sr=8-4/ref=pd_ka_4/104-7475717-5520728?v=glance&s=books&n=507846

Mosby's Comprehensive Review of Dental Hygiene

http://www.amazon.com/exec/obidos/tg/detail/-/0323013163/qid=1089297271/sr=8-2/ref=pd_ka_2/104-7475717-5520728?v=glance&s=books&n=507846

These guides are THE best comprehensive coursework guides to the licensure exams. If you want to spend a couple months in preparation to squeeze every last drop out of your score, buy these books!

Special Report- Review Tables and Images

Eruption Dates for Permanent Teeth

Tooth	Lower	Upper
Central Incisor	6 - 7 years	7 - 8 years
Lateral Incisor	7 - 8 years	8 - 9 years
Canine	9 - 10 years	11 - 12 years
1st Premolar	10 - 12 years	10 -11 years
2nd Premolar	11 - 12 years	10 - 12 years
1st Molar	6 - 7 years	6 - 7 years
2nd Molar	11 - 13 years	12 - 13 years
3rd Molar	17 - 21 years	17 - 21 years

Baby Teeth Eruption Dates

Tooth	Lower	Upper
Central Incisor	6 1/2 months	7 1/2 months
Lateral Incisor	7 months	8 months
First Molar	12 - 16 months	12 - 16 months
Canine	16 - 20 months	16 - 20 months
Second Molar	20 - 30 months	20 - 30 months

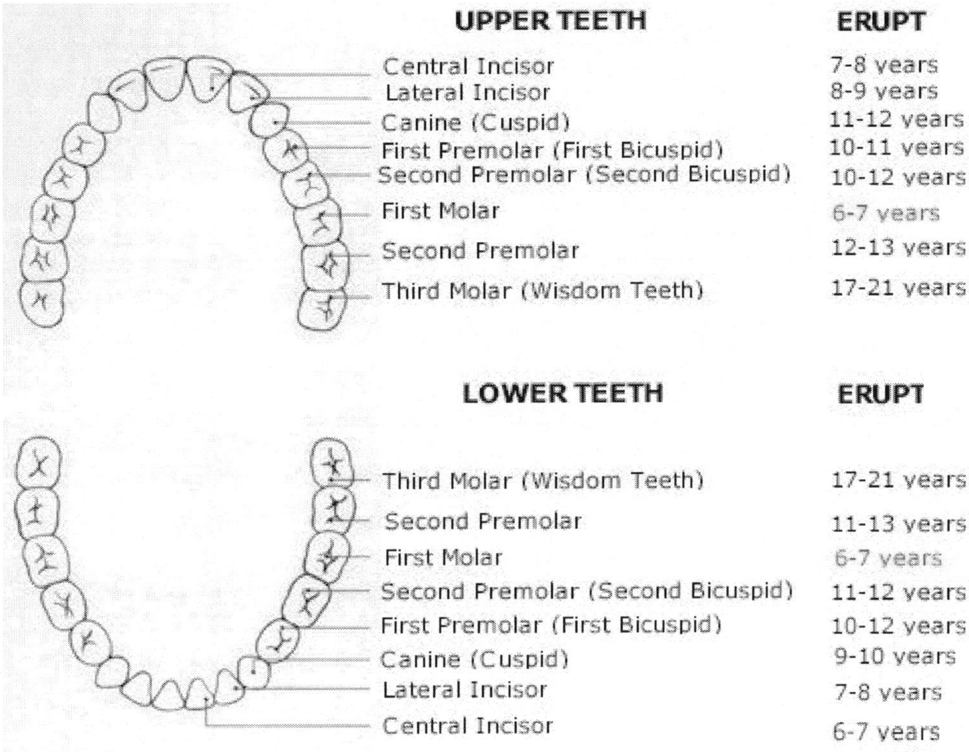

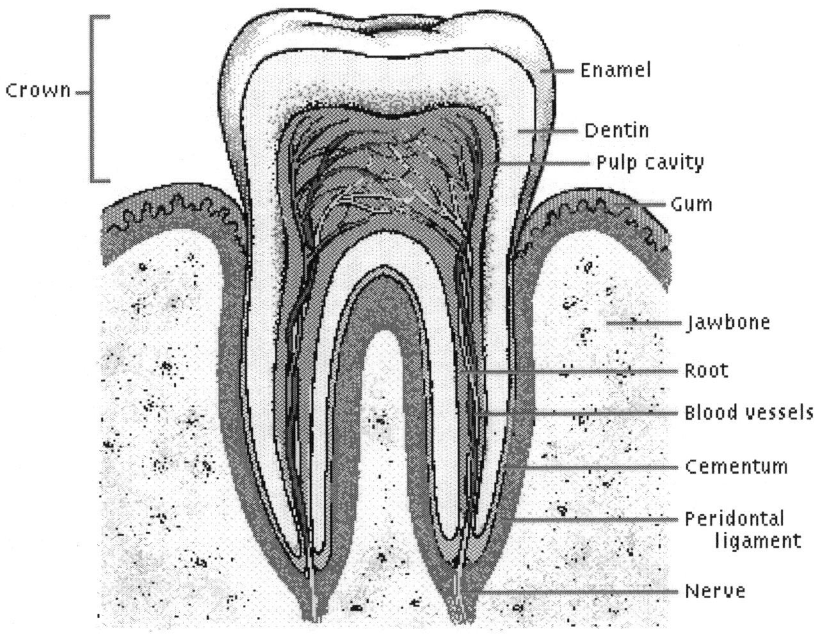

Lateral View

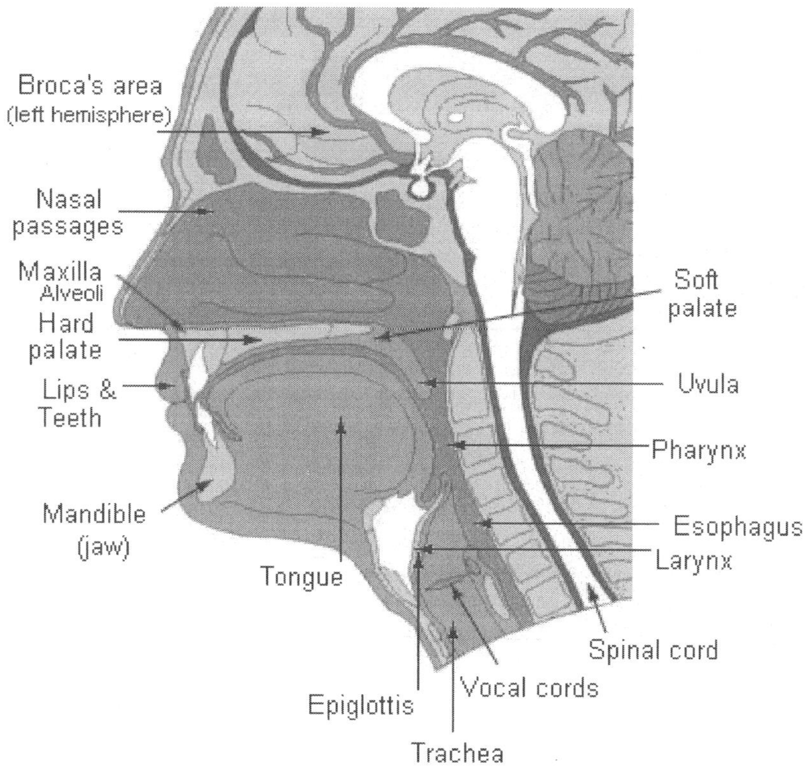

Skull Anatomy

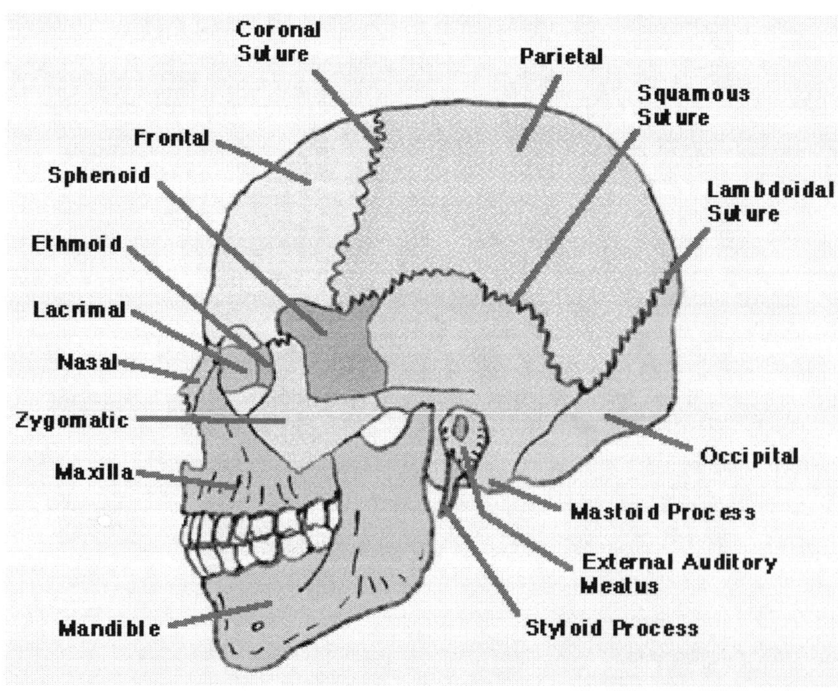

S.mutans Role in Plaque Formation

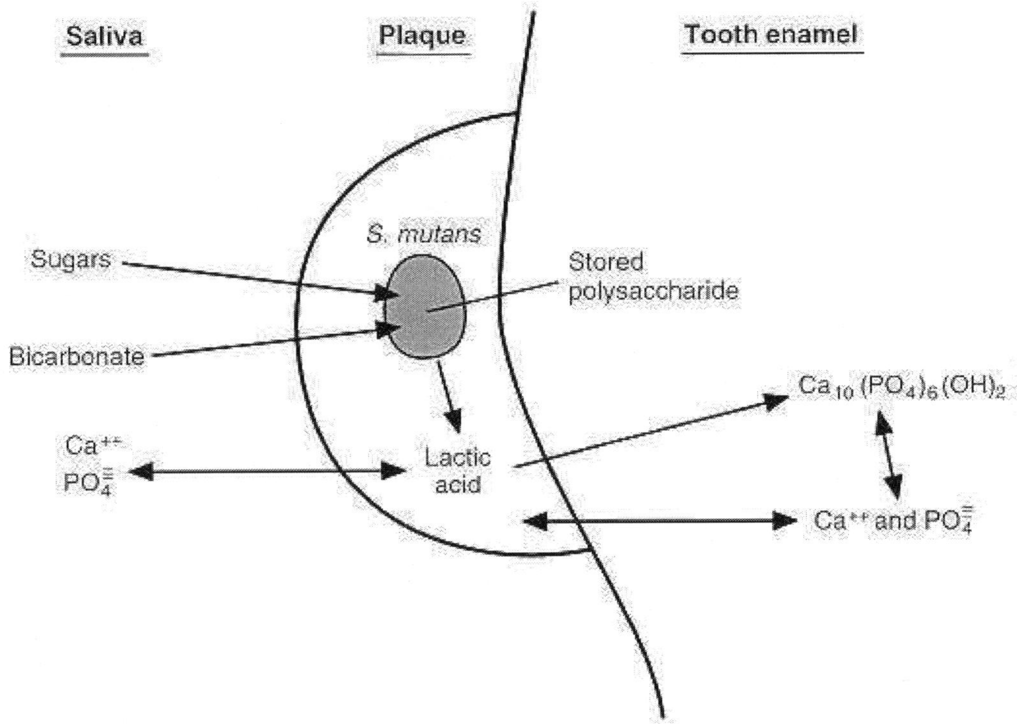

Role of Fluoride

1. Tooth mineral is made less soluble by the formation of fluorapatite during development

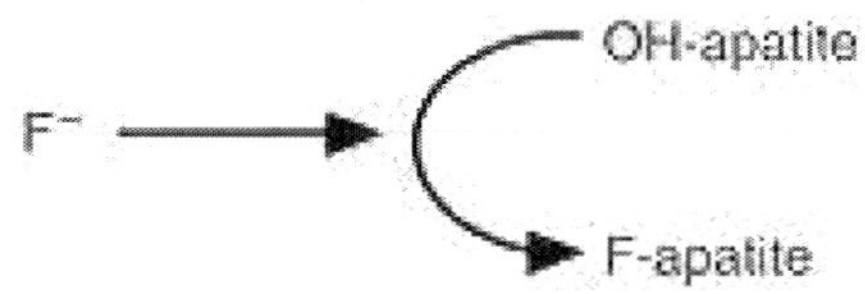

2. Fluoride in saliva and plaque promotes remineralization of tooth surface after tooth eruption

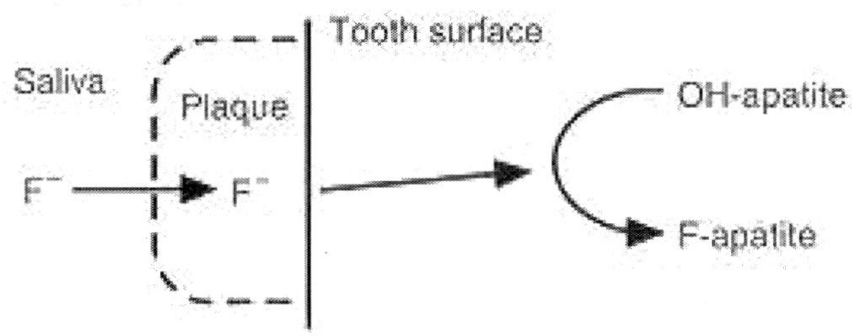

3. Fluoride in plaque enters bacterial cells, especially at low pH, and inhibits enolase, thereby reducing acid production in plaque.

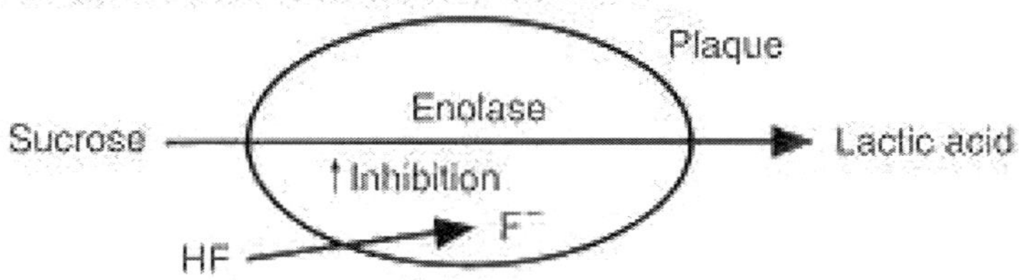

Bonus Report – Dental Organizations

Academy for Sports Dentistry - Organization providing info and ideas for protection from sports related mouth injuries.

Academy of General Dentistry - Organization Committed to ongoing continuing education for Dentists.

Academy of Interdisciplinary Dentofacial Therapy - A comprehensive approach to patient care.

Academy of Laser Dentistry - Organization committed to laser education and research in Dentistry.

Academy of Osseointegration - Organization committed to furthering the education and research concerning implant dentistry.

Alpha Omega International Dental Fraternity - International group offering lectures, study groups, continuing education.

American Academy of Cosmetic Dentistry - Dedicated to advancing the Art and Science of Cosmetic Dentistry.

American Academy of Dental Hygiene - Fostering education and research in the field of dental hygiene.

American Academy of Dental Practice Administration - Committed to providing practice management information for dentists.

American Academy of Esthetic Dentistry - Promoting the integration of esthetics into the total spectrum of oral health care.

American Academy of Fixed Prosthodontics - Committed to competency in research and practice of crown and bridge prosthodontics.

American Academy of Implant Dentistry - Advancing the practice of Implant Dentistry through education and credentialing.

American Academy of Implant Prosthodontics - Providing ongoing training and support for excellence in Implant Dentistry.

American Academy of Maxillofacial Prosthetics - Dedicated to prosthetic correction and management of maxillofacial defects.

American Academy of Orofacial Pain - Includes a detailed tutorial about TMD and orofacial pain.

American Academy of Pediatric Dentistry - Oral health care for infants, children and adolescents.

American Academy of Periodontology - Committed to advancing the periodontal health of the public.

American Academy of Restorative Dentistry - The mission of the Academy is to promote the improvement of the health of the public, and the quality of the art and science of restorative dentistry.

American Association for Dental Research - To represent and support the oral health research community.

American Association for Dental Research - Chicago Section - An organization committed to supporting dental research..

American Association of Dental Schools - All U.S. and Canadian Dental Schools and continuing education programs.

American Association of Endodontists - Promoting research and ideas to encourage excellence in endodontics.

American Association of Oral and Maxillofacial Surgeons - Organization of maxillofacial surgeons.

American Association of Oral Biologists - An independent association supporting education, research and clinical practice in the discipline of Oral Biology.

American Association of Orthodontists - Association committed to educating the public and advancing the art of orthodontics.

American Association of Public Health Dentistry - Supporting and promoting public education and awareness of oral health care.

American Board of Forensic Odontology - The Board that sets the standards for dentists practicing forensic odontology.

American Cleft Palate-Craniofacial Association - Research and education for specialists and families of individuals with cleft palate.

American College of Dentists - Organization of leaders in Dentistry who have made major contributions to dentistry.

American College of Forensic Examiners - Providing education and training for forensic examinations.

American College of Prosthodontics - Promoting the high quality care of prosthodontic patients.

American Dental Assistants Association - To promote the dental assisting profession and promote education and legislation to enhance the delivery of quality denatl health care.
American Dental Association - The ADA is the leading dental site for professionals and consumer info.
American Dental Hygienists Association - Providing info to hygienists and to the public.
American Dental Society of Anesthesiology - Organization committed to education and high standards for anesthesiology and pain control.

Bonus Report – Guidelines for Universal Precautions

Universal precautions are precautions taken to avoid contracting various diseases and preventing the spread of disease to those who have compromised immunity. Some of these diseases include human immunodeficiency virus (HIV), acquired immunodeficiency syndrome (AIDS), and hepatitis B (HBV). Universal precautions are needed since many diseases do not display signs or symptoms in their early stages. Universal precautions mean to treat all body fluids/ substances as if they were contaminated. These body fluids include but are not limited to the following blood, semen, vaginal secretions, breast milk, amniotic fluid, feces, urine, peritoneal fluid, synovial fluid, cerebrospinal fluid, secretions from the nasal and oral cavities, and lacrimal and sweat gland excretions. This means that universal precautions should be used with all patients.

1. A shield for the eyes and face must be used if there is a possibility of splashes from blood and body fluids.
2. If possibility of blood or body fluids being splashed on clothing, you must wear a plastic apron.
3. Gloves must be worn if you could possibly come in contact with blood or body fluids. They are also needed if you are going to touch something that may have come in contact with blood or body fluids.
4. Hands must be washed even if you were wearing gloves. Hands must be washed and gloves must be changed between patients. Wash hands with at a dime size amount of soap and warm water for about 30 seconds. Singing "Mary had a little lamb" is approximately 30 seconds.
5. Blood and body fluid spills must be cleansed and disinfected using a solution of one part bleach to 10 parts water or your hospital's accepted method.
6. Used needles must be separated from clean needles. Throw both the needle and the syringe away in the sharps' container. The sharps' container is made of puncture proof material.
7. Take extra care in performing high-risk activities that include puncturing the skin and cutting the skin.

Special precautions must be taken to dispose of biomedical waste. Biomedical waste includes but is not limited to the following: laboratory waste, pathology waste, liquid waste from suction, all sharp object, bladder catheters, chest tubes, IV tubes, and drainage containers. Biomedical waste is removed from a facility by trained biomedical waste disposers.

The health care professional is legally and ethically responsible for adhering to universal precautions. They may prevent you from contracting a fatal disease or from a patient contracting a disease from you that could be deadly.

CPR Review/Cheat Sheet

Topic	New Guidelines
Conscious Choking	5 back blows, then 5 abdominal thrusts- adult/child
Unconscious Choking	5 chest compressions, look, 2 breaths-adult/child/infant
Rescue Breaths	Normal Breath given over 1 second until chest rises
Chest Compressions to Ventilation Ratios (Single Rescuer)	30:2 – Adult/Child/Infant
Chest Compressions to Ventilation Ratios (Two Rescuer)	30:2 – Adult 15:2 – Child/Infant
Chest Compression rate	About 100/minute – Adult/Child/Infant
Chest Compression Land marking Method	Simplified approach – center of the chest – Adult/Child 2 or 3 fingers, just below the nipple line at the center of the chest - Infant
AED	1 shock, then 2 minutes (or 5 cycles) of CPR
Anaphylaxis	Assist person with use of prescribed auto injector
Asthma	Assist person with use of prescribed inhaler

- Check the scene
- Check for responsiveness – ask, "Are you OK?"
- Adult - call 911, then administer CPR
- Child/Infant – administer CPR for 5 cycles, then call 911
- Open victim's airway and check for breathing – look, listen, and feel for 5 - 10 seconds
- Two rescue breaths should be given, 1 second each, and should produce a visible chest rise
- If the air does not go in, reposition and try 2 breaths again
- Check victim's pulse – chest compressions are recommended if an infant or child has a rate less than 60 per minute with signs of poor perfusion.
- Begin 30 compressions to 2 breaths at a rate of 1 breath every 5 seconds for Adult; 1 breath every 3 seconds for child/infant
- Continue 30:2 ratio until victim moves, AED is brought to the scene, or professional help arrives

AED

- ADULT/ Child over 8 years old - use Adult pads

- Child 1-8 years old – use Child pads or use Adult pads by placing one on the chest and one on the back of the child
- Infant under 1 year of age - AED not recommended

Special Report: Additional Bonus Material

Due to our efforts to try to keep this book to a manageable length, we've created a link that will give you access to all of your additional bonus material.

Please visit http://www.mo-media.com/nbdhe/bonuses to access the information.